BECOMING

THE

VISION

Published and distributed by Merack Publishing
Jackson, USA
www.merackpublishing.com

Library of Congress Control Number: 2025909971
Peddle, Angela
*Becoming the Vision: The Transformational Power of Vision to Heal, Awaken, and
Become Who You Were Meant to Be*

ISBN
Paperback 978-1-964421-11-7
eBook 978-1-964421-12-4

BECOMING

THE

VISION

The Transformational Power of Vision to Heal,
Awaken, and Become Who You Were Meant to Be

ANGELA PEDDLE

To every person who has ever felt unseen, unheard, or misunderstood—this book is for you. May it remind you that vision is more than eyesight. It's a way of feeling safe in the world. A way of understanding who you are. A way of coming home to yourself.

CONTENTS

DEAR READER,

Before we begin, I want to tell you something true. I almost didn't write this. Not because I didn't feel called—but because I didn't feel *qualified*.

You see, I was trained to be precise. Clinical. Measurable. To stay in my lane, speak in peer-reviewed terms, and never say too much. But what I witnessed in my practice . . . broke all of that.

I watched children say their first words with a lens that wasn't "strong enough to matter."

I saw concussion survivors drop their shoulders and cry from one tint of light.

I watched regulated breath return to trauma survivors who hadn't exhaled in years.

And none of that was in the textbooks.

For a long time, I tried to keep the magic quiet. To make it sound more acceptable. To translate what I knew into the language of data, evidence, and linear logic. But eventually, something in me broke. Or maybe . . . opened.

And I realized: The truth I carry didn't come from textbooks. It came from *every soul I've sat with*.

From the parents who were told "everything looks fine," but knew in their gut something was off.

From the children who couldn't read the chart but could read the *room* with laser precision.

From my own body, which stopped lighting up in conventional practice and started pulsing with truth when I stepped into what I *knew* but couldn't yet prove.

So this book? It's not about fixing your eyes.

It's about coming home to the way you were always meant to see.

It will weave together science, story, soul, and safety. It might challenge what you've been taught.

It might wake something in you you've buried. And it might give you language for the thing you've always *felt* . . . but never knew how to name.

I don't pretend to have all the answers. But I *do* have the pattern. The one I've been tracing through thousands of patients, hundreds of stories, and decades of remembering.

I'm not here to convince you. I'm here to invite you.

To see through a new lens.

To remember what your vision *really is*.

To begin a process that is both neurological . . . and sacred.

I wrote this for you. But I also wrote it to finally tell the truth.

So let's begin—together.

With light,
Angela Noelle Peddle

INTRODUCTION

The Inner Lens — Remembering How to See

Before you read another word, I want you to know this: you already hold the answers. You already have the wisdom. My job isn't to give you anything you don't already possess. My job is to help you remember.

This book is about vision—but not only the kind that involves the eyes. It's about the vision that lives beneath perception. The kind that sees with the body. With the soul. With the heart that has been aching for clarity, connection, and the freedom to fully show up in this life.

I've spent my whole career helping people see. And yet, what I've come to understand is this: the most powerful breakthroughs don't happen through lenses, or therapy rooms, or treatment plans. They happen when we meet the unseen. The subconscious patterns. The emotional imprints. What sits behind the eyes.

And when we finally stop trying to fix people . . . and instead begin to witness them . . . that's when the real vision returns. Not just the clinical kind, but the soul-led kind. The kind that helps us feel alive again. The kind that connects the brain, the body, the heart, and something far greater than logic.

This isn't only a book about vision. This is a map back to wholeness—through the doorway of sight.

You may be a practitioner. A parent. A seeker. A survivor. You may be exhausted from trying to find answers.

Let this be your permission to soften. Let this be a mirror for your brilliance. Let this be a return to your inner lens—the one that's always known.

Welcome.

I'm so glad you're here.

PREFACE

Under the Rock, A New Shell

I left optometry school glowing. I had trained at the Pennsylvania College of Optometry, drawn there for their rare advanced pediatric track. As a Canadian, this program was my golden thread—to weave my passion for pediatrics and eye care into one amazing calling.

I loved it. I thrived. I absorbed everything. As I went deeper into pediatrics, I learned about vision therapy—in its classical form—and it felt like coming home.

Then I got accepted into my dream residency at SUNY College of Optometry in New York City—focused on functional rehabilitation, a more behavioral approach to vision therapy—and this lit an even deeper fire in me. When students would ask me later in life if they should pursue a residency, I have always said that it was the single most important choice I made for my career.

I returned to Canada after my residency filled with purpose. I was ready to bring this powerful work home.

And then I hit the wall.

Not a gentle resistance. A brick wall of skepticism, dismissal, and shaming.

I hadn't even cultivated my more advanced neuro-cognitive work yet. I was still practicing a more classical model of vision therapy, and I was excited to help others with what I knew. But just the phrase "vision therapy" was enough to be labeled.

Vision therapy? Snake oil.

You're in it for the money.

There's no evidence. Children's brains aren't neuroplastic after the age of nine. Haven't you read the studies?

I was crushed.

But here's what those people don't know:

Vision therapy is not eye exercises. It is not a gimmick. It is not a last resort.

It is a neuroplastic process that helps rewire how the brain and body use visual information. At any age.

It restores balance, depth, clarity, connection—not just to the world, but to oneself.

And I knew what I had seen. I had seen children see depth for the first time. Adults walk again. Teens reclaim their confidence.

But no one wanted to hear it. I wasn't welcome in my own profession.

So I cried. I doubted. I tried to shrink.

And then I remembered the story of a lobster that I heard once.

Do you know how a lobster grows? When it becomes uncomfortable in its shell, it crawls under a rock, sheds its old armor, and grows a new one.

Their stimulus for growth is discomfort.

And I realized: I wasn't being pushed out. I was being called through. So I stopped trying to fit in. And I started to build.

I founded Vision Therapy Canada.

What started as a small circle of dreamers grew into a national organization with over 400 members within only a few years. I had found my tribe, and we were on fire.

We educated the public. We trained practitioners.

We ruffled feathers. I got letters. Legal threats.

But I had outgrown the old shell. I wasn't defending my work anymore. I was living it.

And that . . . that was the beginning of this book.

A Note on the
Micro-Healing Invitations

Throughout this book, you'll find something called a *Micro-Healing Invitation* at the end of each chapter. These are not summaries or action steps in the traditional sense. They are moments—small but powerful invitations to integrate what you've just read, not only with your mind but with your body, your breath, and your nervous system.

Each Micro-Healing is grounded in neuroscience, yet gentle in spirit. They're designed to spark self-regulation, deepen emotional awareness, and bring vision back into relationship with the whole self.

You don't need to "do" them all. Let your system guide you. Some may feel like quiet pauses. Others, like catalysts.

They are here to help you not just learn but experience the Neuro-Integrative Vision Model in real time.

Because transformation doesn't happen through information alone.

It happens when we allow the body to remember, the heart to feel, and the self to be seen.

1

How You See
Is How You Live

A Truth That Changes Everything

We've been taught to believe that vision is just eyesight. That 20/20 means "all is well." If we can read the eye chart, see clearly, and don't need glasses, then our visual system must be healthy. But what if that definition is not only limited—it's actually the thing holding us back?

Vision is not just clarity. It isn't a static score or a test result. It isn't something that happens only in the eyes. Vision is a dynamic, neuro-plastic process that's shaped by—and actively shapes—your brain, your body, your breath, your emotions, and your relationships. It influences far more than clarity. It shapes your posture, your sense of orientation in space, your depth perception, your balance, your ability to feel safe in a room, and your perception of what's real and what isn't.

It affects how you navigate light, crowds, movement, and the unknown. It touches how you learn, how you focus, how you relate to others—and how you feel about yourself. This isn't just about eyesight. This is about *how you experience the world*. And yet, even that explanation doesn't fully capture what I've witnessed in the clinical room. There's a deeper layer—one that traditional models can't quite explain, but that I've learned to recognize through the nervous system, the emotional body, and the subconscious field.

Because here's the truth that changes everything: vision is perception. And perception is deeply personal. It is not neutral. It is not passive. It is filtered through your history, your nervous system, your beliefs, your traumas, and your physiology. This is why two people can look at the exact same image and have completely different emotional, physiological, and behavioral responses. Vision is not simply about receiving light. It is about interpreting reality.

Perception Is the Lens Between You and the World

You don't see with your eyes. You see with your brain. With your nervous system. With the subconscious filter shaped by your life experience. And when that filter is burdened with old patterns or protective adaptations, the world itself begins to feel unfamiliar—fragmented, unsafe, or overwhelming.

Your eyes act, as a very simple analogy, as the camera—but it is your brain that edits the image. And if that internal editor has been shaped by fear, trauma, suppression, or chronic stress, the world you see may appear distorted, overwhelming, fragmented, or unsafe.

People with visual dysfunction aren't simply "seeing differently" in the optical sense. They are *living differently*. Their posture changes. Their breathing patterns shift. They struggle to read not because they lack intelligence, but because their system is unable to remain regulated long enough to process the visual input. They avoid bright lights because their system is already overstimulated. They shut down in classrooms, offices, and social settings—not because they're disinterested, but because their perceptual system can't find grounding.

And if we keep treating this as a "vision problem," we'll continue to miss the deeper point. We'll keep addressing symptoms without touching the roots—the emotional imprints, inherited responses, and energetic contractions that quietly shape how vision operates beneath the surface.

The Visual System Is Emotional

More than 50% of the brain is involved in visual processing. That's not philosophy—that's neuroscience. But what often goes unspoken, even in professional circles, is that vision is deeply entwined with the limbic system—the part of the brain that governs emotion, memory, and survival.

What this means is that visual input isn't just processed logically. It's processed emotionally.

In other words, *the way you see is influenced by how you feel.* And how you feel, in turn, is influenced by the way you see.

This is why some children act out in visually chaotic classrooms.

Why trauma survivors experience tunnel vision or hypersensitivity to light.

Why individuals recovering from concussion often say the world feels "off," "too much," or "not real."

Why some patients cry the moment they try on a lens that feels inexplicably *right*—before they even understand what changed.

They're not reacting to the letters on a wall. They're reacting to the *felt experience* of how their nervous system is interpreting what they see. And that interpretation is shaped by far more than eye movements or refractive status. It is shaped by stored emotion, subconscious beliefs, and the body's unspoken memories.

And that . . . is everything.

Vision Is the Forgotten Sense of the Subconscious

We talk about gut feelings.

We explore somatic trauma, vagus nerve healing, and the intelligence of the body.

But we often forget that vision is the most dominant sensory input in most people's lives.

It is fast. It is constant. It is emotionally loaded. And yet, we rarely consider how our visual system has been shaped by our history—by our experiences, our beliefs, our sense of safety or danger. What if vision holds not only perception—but protection? And what if it also holds the key to healing beyond what we've known?

What if vision is not just an input . . . but a mirror?

What if it's the fastest access point we have to the subconscious?

Because when you look through a lens shaped by the past, you continue to recreate that past—over and over again. But when the visual system is given the opportunity to reorganize—to repattern, rewire, and *remember*—something remarkable happens.

The system doesn't just see differently.

It starts to feel safe. And when safety returns . . . healing begins. This is where my work began to evolve: where traditional lens prescribing met something more—something intuitive, integrative, and alive.

This isn't a metaphor.

This is neurology.

This is embodied science.

This is the missing link.

This Is the Work of Remembering

When you begin to understand how your perception has been shaped—by pain, by pattern, by survival—you begin to gain the power to reshape it.

This is the essence of my **Neuro-Integrative Vision Model.** Not to fix your eyes. But to restore your internal lens. To meet the places where vision and emotion overlap. Where a lens becomes a language—and a prescription becomes a permission slip for the nervous system to return to itself.

To help you identify where your system has dimmed or distorted your vision to protect you . . . and to gently invite it back toward clarity, integration, and presence.

Because the way you see . . . is the way you live. And when you change how you see . . .

You begin to change *everything*.

Let's begin.

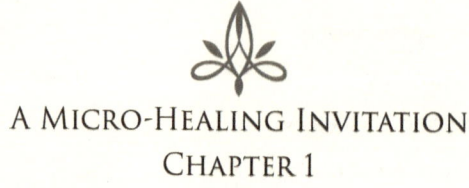

A MICRO-HEALING INVITATION
CHAPTER 1

Seeing Beneath the Surface

Your brain processes far more than you're consciously aware of. Much of what we see—what we notice, filter, or ignore—happens before thought. This is not a flaw. It's a feature of your adaptive, efficient nervous system.

Take a moment now to engage with it more deliberately.

Place a hand gently over your chest or belly—wherever you feel breath most easily. Inhale through your nose for a count of four. Exhale slowly through your mouth for a count of six.

Then ask:

- What area of my life am I operating on autopilot?

- Where might deeper perception be possible?

Don't try to force an answer. Let your body respond first.

A sigh. A sensation. A small shift in attention.

That is perception reorganizing itself. Let it happen.

2

THE MODELS
WE'VE OUTGROWN

Breaking the Frame So We Can Truly See

We are taught to trust models. They give us structure. They offer clarity in a sea of complexity—something to hold onto when things feel uncertain or vast. They help us categorize what we observe, name what we sense, and make clinical decisions with greater precision. But at their core, models are scaffolds—tools for understanding, not permanent truths. They help us build something. But eventually, we outgrow the very thing that once gave us form.

They are meant to evolve. Science teaches us this. Life demands it.

And in the field of vision science, we are standing at that edge now. Not because the models have failed—but because our patients are inviting us into more than the models were built to hold.

The definitions we've inherited—what vision is, how it develops, and how it should be treated—have become too small to hold what we are actually seeing unfold in real patients, in real systems, in real life. We are witnessing outcomes and transformations that do not fit within the boxes we've been taught.

Sometimes, these insights arrive before the literature does. In practice, we meet patterns that science has not yet named. We feel shifts in the nervous system that aren't easily explained by traditional mechanisms. We prescribe lenses that shouldn't make a difference— but do. Profoundly.

We sense emotional releases. We notice breath patterns change. We witness presence returning to a body that had once dissociated from space. And quietly, something in us begins to ask—what else is happening here?

This is where innovation begins. Not in peer-reviewed journals—but in the presence of patients. In the hands of practitioners who are willing to see beyond the model, while still honoring what the model once offered.

We must also acknowledge a quiet truth: sometimes, those who have practiced the longest may unknowingly carry models that no longer match the moment. Not because they lack skill, but because science evolves faster than systems of education—and far faster than comfort allows.

So we are being asked to do something difficult, but essential: we must evolve the model.

Not because the older ones were wrong. But because they were never meant to be the final destination. They were stepping stones that brought us here—beautiful, brilliant, and incomplete.

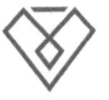

The Living Model in the Room

Not long ago, I worked with a woman who had sustained a traumatic brain injury in a motor vehicle accident. By the time she reached me, years had passed since the incident. Her balance was still severely impaired. She walked cautiously, with a wide, robotic gait. Her movements were stiff, effortful, disconnected from the fluid grace she once knew.

She had done the work. Weeks of physiotherapy. Exercises. Progress had been made. But something was still missing— something no one could name. "Post-concussion syndrome," they said. "You should learn to accept your new normal."

She couldn't accept that she was forever relegated to this new "normal," and days of painstaking online research landed her in my office. She described to me her overwhelming discomfort in everyday situations: the fluorescent lights of grocery stores, the movement of people on a sidewalk, even the narrowness of a hallway. Her body no longer felt like her own. Her vestibular system, her visual system, and her somatic awareness were trying to speak—but no one had listened in the language they were using.

When I assessed her, I didn't just check her acuity or eye movements. I observed how her system moved through space. I looked at how her nervous system held posture. How her steps *shifted during the Fakuda stepping test. How her tandem walk revealed subtle, subconscious hesitations. Her brain no longer had a clear map of where her body was in relation to the room around her. Her relationship to space—and to gravity—was fragmented.*

So I introduced something simple yet highly intentional: a spatially yoked prism, a lens that shifts space gently. Not to correct a refractive error. Not to "sharpen" her sight. But to help her nervous system reclaim its orientation in space. Her eyes weren't giving her system stable information, so her system acted unstable.

She put the lenses on and took a single step.

It was smooth.

Her gait softened. Her posture adjusted. Her body stood taller, but with less effort. Her shoulders dropped. Her facial muscles relaxed. She blinked—slowly, with ease. And then . . . she smiled.

That smile wasn't just relief. It was recognition. For the first time since the accident, she could feel where her body ended and the world began. Her spatial boundaries returned. And that single shift—perceptual and somatic—changed everything. What we had accessed wasn't just visual function—it was her internal orientation system. Something deeper. Something alive beneath the traditional map of vision science.

Through vision, she returned home to herself.

Why We Create Models in the First Place

When something as vast and complex as vision needs to be understood, we naturally try to break it into parts. We look for patterns. We name what we can see. We categorize what we can measure. This is how every model begins.

Before diving into the more widely accepted models of vision, we must pause to acknowledge the earliest—and perhaps most visionary—framework in the behavioral optometry field: Skeffington's Four Circles. Conceived in the mid-twentieth century, this model didn't just describe vision in terms of optics or mechanics. It described it as an emergent process—born from the interplay of four interconnected systems: anti-gravity (posture and body awareness), centering (attention and orientation), identification (recognition and meaning-making), and speech-auditory (communication and response).[1,2]

Skeffington was not merely defining how the eyes work. He was articulating how vision arises from the totality of human experience.

Yet, despite its brilliance, the Four Circles model was seen by some as too abstract, too philosophical, too "out there" to be embraced by the mainstream. As the field of optometry began aligning more closely with evidence-based, biomedical paradigms, Skeffington's ideas were gradually pushed to the margins—kept alive only by a small but devoted group of behavioral and developmental optometrists who understood the model's depth.

Ironically, as neuroscience has advanced and begun validating many of Skeffington's claims—about the embodied, perceptual, and emotional nature of vision—his model feels more relevant

1   Schmitt, E. P. (2005). A.M. Skeffington: Father of Behavioral Optometry. Santa Ana, CA: Optometric Extension Program Foundation.
2   Press, L. J. (1997). Applied concepts in vision therapy. St. Louis, MO: Mosby.

than ever. It serves as a powerful reminder that some frameworks are simply ahead of their time. And that sometimes, in the rush to be scientific, we lose sight of the systems-level wisdom that sees the whole person—not just the eyes.

As optometry sought to define itself more concretely within the medical sciences, a shift occurred. The profession leaned into the precision and reliability of measurable outcomes, and what emerged was a classical model of vision. This model provided clarity and order. It focused on ocular health, refractive error, and the structural components of the visual system—what could be seen, tested, and quantified.

In many ways, this model helped ground the profession in credibility. It allowed us to identify pathology, diagnose refractive conditions, and restore 20/20 acuity. But its lens was narrow. It treated the eyes as isolated organs and vision as a mechanical process—light in, image formed, interpretation presumed. It missed the dynamic interplay between vision and body, vision and brain, vision and experience.

Still, this model served an essential purpose. It gave us structure—something to build upon.

And so, as our understanding of vision deepened—especially through the growing field of vision therapy—we continued to revise and refine our frameworks. New layers of complexity emerged. We began to see that clarity alone was not enough. That binocular dysfunction, perceptual delays, and learning challenges required a broader lens.

This led to the development of three core models that have shaped the field to this day:

- The Classical Structural Model
- The Visual Functional Model
- The Neuro-Cognitive Model

Each of these models has brought profound value. Each marked a turning point in how we understand and treat vision. They have moved our profession forward in essential ways. But now, we are beginning to feel their limits. We are meeting patients whose experiences don't fully fit within any of them. We are hearing questions—both in our clinics and in our own hearts—that no longer have clear answers within the old frames.

And that is often the sign: not of failure, but of evolution.

The Classical Structural Model

"The eyes are organs. Fix the organ, restore the function."

This is the model every optometrist is trained in first—and, for many, the only model they ever work from. It's the foundation of traditional optometry, based on anatomy, optics, and ocular health.

It teaches us how to assess refraction, ocular motility, convergence, and accommodation. It guides us in diagnosing and treating myopia, hyperopia, astigmatism, amblyopia, and ocular disease. It's essential. Without this knowledge, we couldn't recognize retinal detachments, optic nerve disease, or visual field loss due to stroke.

This model focuses on the eyes as isolated systems—organs that can be tested, measured, and corrected. It operates within a medical framework: if something is broken, diagnose and fix it. If the structure is intact, the function must be fine.

And here's the core problem with that logic: if a patient's symptoms don't match a visible structural issue, they're often told nothing is wrong.

This is where thousands of patients fall through the cracks.

In this model, if a child passes a visual acuity test, they're considered "fine"—even if they complain of reading fatigue, or trouble focusing in class. If an adult's eye exam is normal, but they report light sensitivity, dizziness, or visual overwhelm, they're often dismissed—or worse, sent home with the suggestion that it's "just stress" or "all in their head."

But what if it's in their perception? What if their system is speaking through symptoms we haven't been trained to listen for?

That's where the limitations of this structural model end—and the need for the next model begins.

The Visual Functional Model

"Vision is learned. Vision develops. Let's help it mature."

This model takes us deeper. It's primarily used by optometrists who specialize in vision therapy and rehabilitation—those who understand that vision is not just a passive process, but an active, trainable, and adaptive one.

In the Visual Functional Model, vision is a learned skill that develops through movement, experience, and integration. It's tied to motor coordination, spatial awareness, posture, balance, and bilateral body organization. This model helps us understand that visual problems can arise even when the eyes are structurally healthy—because the system is not integrated.

We begin to work with concepts like:

- Visual-motor integration
- Eye-hand coordination
- Near-point stress
- Vestibulo-ocular reflexes
- Primitive reflex retention
- Laterality and directionality
- Core stability and peripheral awareness

This is where we start working with developmental delays, convergence insufficiency, postural distortions, and the impacts of early trauma or sensory deprivation on vision.

The Functional Model also considers how vision interacts with other sensory systems—especially the vestibular, tactile, and proprioceptive systems. Practitioners trained in this model often collaborate with occupational therapists, speech language pathologists, and other somatic practitioners.

But here's the truth: most traditional optometrists don't work here. They weren't trained to see vision this way.

And because it challenges the medical model of quick fixes, some dismiss it entirely.

Even those who enter this realm often stop at the behavioral level—they focus on training visual efficiency and skills without fully exploring what drives perception beneath the surface.

This is where we begin to feel the limitations again.

Because even this model struggles to account for what lives beneath behavior. What about the subtle dissociation that occurs when a child avoids looking directly at a parent after early trauma? Or the shoulders that won't drop, no matter how integrated the vestibular system becomes?

The Neuro-Cognitive Model

"Vision is brain-driven. Let's understand the neurology."

This model, taken to the next level by visionary Dr. Robert Sanet, takes us into the brain. It reframes vision not as a function of the eyes, but as a complex, multi-stream processing system involving over 50% of the cerebral cortex.

Note: The neuroanatomical and functional pathways described here are supported by peer-reviewed neuroscience research, including foundational work on the dorsal/ventral streams (Ungerleider & Mishkin, 1982), the pulvinar's role in attention (Saalmann & Kastner, 2011), and the superior colliculus in reflexive gaze and integration (May, 2006). For a full list of sources, see References on page 161.

We learn about:

The Dorsal Stream

Often called the "where" pathway, the dorsal stream begins in the primary visual cortex and projects upward into the parietal lobes. It is responsible for spatial orientation, depth perception, and motion tracking. This pathway tells us where things are in space—not just external objects, but our own body in relation to the world. It helps us maintain midline awareness, navigate through crowded environments, and coordinate movement. When the dorsal stream is disrupted, people often feel clumsy, disoriented, or "not grounded." They may bump into doorways, struggle with balance, or feel unsafe in visually complex settings. This stream is essential for body mapping and movement through space.

The Ventral Stream

Known as the "what" pathway, the ventral stream also originates in the visual cortex but travels downward into the temporal lobes. It is responsible for recognizing and assigning meaning to what we see—faces, objects, symbols, words. This is the pathway that allows a child to recognize their parent's face, or an adult to read and comprehend text. When the ventral stream is disrupted, a person may have difficulty identifying visual details, recognizing facial expressions, or attaching emotional significance to visual input. It's the stream of meaning-making—and when it's overwhelmed, even a familiar environment can feel unrecognizable. This "what" pathway is for object recognition, facial perception, and meaning.

The Pulvinar Nucleus

The pulvinar is a lesser-known but critically important part of the thalamus—a hub that filters visual information before it reaches conscious awareness. It acts like a gatekeeper, helping the brain prioritize what to focus on. It is especially sensitive to threat-related stimuli and is heavily involved in subconscious visual attention. When the pulvinar is overactive or dysregulated, it can lead to hypervigilance, poor visual filtering, or difficulty maintaining focus in visually stimulating environments. For trauma survivors or post-concussion patients, this structure often plays a key role in light sensitivity and environmental overwhelm.

The Superior Colliculus

The superior colliculus is part of the midbrain and is involved in rapid, reflexive visual orientation. It coordinates eye movements and head turns in response to sudden changes in the visual field. This is the structure that allows you to instinctively look when something moves out of the corner of your eye. It also plays a role in multisensory integration—blending visual, auditory, and somatic input. When impaired, patients may struggle with saccadic eye movements or tracking, or experience delayed responses to visual stimuli. It can also contribute to "freezing" behaviors in response to visual overwhelm.

The Reticular Activating System (RAS)

The RAS is a network of neurons located in the brainstem that regulates wakefulness, attention, and arousal. It plays a central role in filtering sensory input and modulating alertness—determining whether the system becomes hyper-alert or disengaged. In vision, the RAS helps determine how alert the brain becomes in response to visual input. A poorly modulated RAS can lead to states of hyper-arousal (e.g., light sensitivity, anxiety) or hypoarousal (e.g., fatigue, inattention, fogginess). The visual system and RAS are deeply interconnected, especially in patients with post-concussive symptoms or sensory processing challenges.

The Parietal Lobe

The parietal lobes serve as a critical integration center for sensory information related to touch, proprioception, and spatial awareness. They play a key role in helping the brain construct a three-dimensional map of the world—and of the body's position within it. This is where vision and movement meet. When the parietal lobes are underactive or disconnected from visual input, patients may experience poor hand-eye coordination, challenges with visual-spatial reasoning, or feel disoriented in space. This area also integrates input from the dorsal stream, making it a crucial region for mobility and postural control.

The Cerebellum

Often associated with balance and coordination, the cerebellum also plays an essential role in visual-motor integration. It helps fine-tune saccades (quick eye movements), smooth pursuits, and visual tracking. It supports rhythm, timing, and anticipatory motor control—all of which influence how we read, move, and engage visually with the world. Dysfunction here often shows up as visual instability during movement, trouble copying from the board, or "jumping lines" while reading. The cerebellum also has emotional connections, making it a quiet but powerful contributor to how we feel when we move through visual space.

For more information about the Neuro-Cognitive Model, please refer to the sources in Appendix A, found on page 157.

In this model, we understand that vision is integrated with attention, memory, emotional processing, and executive function. It is not just a sense—it's an entire network.

This model is what finally helps us explain symptoms like:

- Visual-vestibular mismatch after concussion
- Light sensitivity due to midbrain dysregulation
- Emotional triggers caused by visual input
- Reading challenges with normal intelligence
- Disorientation in busy environments
- Feeling "out of body" in visually complex spaces

It's brilliant. It's powerful. And it brought us closer to the truth. But even this model, as taught today, often stops at dysfunction.

We analyze what pathway is underactive. We chart what area of the brain is "lagging." We look at the system as something to be corrected or optimized.

What's still missing is the felt experience. The emotional resonance. The energetic and intuitive communication happening beneath the level of conscious awareness. This is the place I began exploring through clinical muscle testing, lens-based nervous system mapping, and emotional decoding—not to replace science, but to reveal what it hadn't yet named.

Because before perception becomes measurable . . . it becomes felt.

What All These Models Miss

They stop at the edge of something we've all felt but haven't known how to describe.

That vision is not solely a system of light and movement. It's a system of survival. Of memory. Of intuition. Of soul. None of the traditional models account for the moment when a child cries after putting on the right lenses. Or when a trauma survivor finally steps into space and says, "I feel safe." Or when a patient's voice changes mid-exam because their perception has shifted. Or when someone breathes deeper, stands taller, and reclaims their presence—without knowing why.

What you're witnessing goes beyond function or behavior. This is transformation. You're not discarding the past—you're becoming more because of it.

These models brought us here. They served their purpose. They helped us build understanding and offer real care to thousands. But now it's time for something more.

It's time for a model that doesn't reduce vision to function, but elevates it to what it truly is—a full-body, full-being experience. A model that includes the subconscious. That honors the energetic. That invites the emotional, spiritual, and somatic into the room. A model that allows us to meet patients where they truly are—in the place where vision, emotion, and presence converge.

That's what we'll explore next:

The Neuro-Integrative Vision Model—the next lens. One that doesn't replace what came before . . . but finally brings it all together.

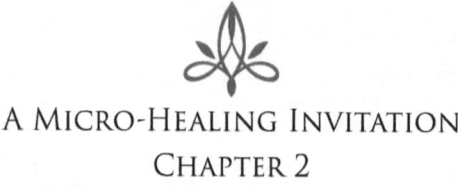

A Micro-Healing Invitation
Chapter 2

The Models We've Outgrown

The brain loves structure. It builds internal models to help us predict, plan, and feel safe in a complex world. But sometimes, the very models that once offered stability can become too small for who we've become.

Take a moment to reflect on one such internal framework— something you were taught, believed, or relied on. A rule, a method, a worldview.

Now ask yourself:

Where in my life or work am I still operating within an outdated model?

Have I experienced something—through my intuition, my relationships, or my professional insights—that no longer fits within that structure?

There's no need to force an answer. Simply notice.

Let your exhale be a soft release of rigidity.

Let your inhale create space for new frameworks to emerge.

Growth doesn't discard the old—it integrates what served and makes room for what's next.

You are allowed to evolve your lens.

You are allowed to see with new eyes.

3

VISION AND THE SUBCONSCIOUS

The Lens That Sees Before You Know You're Looking

THE WALTZ THAT SHATTERED DOUBT

She entered my office leaning on a cane—not by choice, but because her nervous system offered no alternative.

She was seventy years old, radiant in her spirit, and still—against all odds—training for a ballroom dancing competition. She was a professional ballroom dancer her whole life, still competing happily at seventy years old. But after a recent motor vehicle accident on her way to a competition, something in her had changed. Her balance was gone. Her coordination was unpredictable. She walked with effort, every movement cautious and stiff. Her head pounded.

She had tried everything—vestibular therapy, physiotherapy, ophthalmology, occupational therapy, acupuncture. Nothing brought her back to herself.

She was desperate. Not in the dramatic way. But in the quiet, soul-weary way that people become when they're tired of being dismissed. She had seen specialist after specialist, but none could explain what she was feeling. Her brother—a prominent ophthalmologist in another country—told her not to waste her time with me. "What could an optometrist do?" he had asked. And she obliged. For years.

But, now she came anyway, after a trusted occupational therapy colleague of mine convinced her she had nothing to lose.

She sat in my chair and said the words I'll never forget: "You're the last person I'm going to see."

There was something in her tone that shook me. It wasn't casual. It was final. She didn't need data. She needed a miracle.

*As I evaluated her, I noticed something that had been missed. Her body wasn't just unsteady—it was disoriented. Her balance didn't need more strength—it needed **coherence.** Her system wasn't resisting movement—it didn't know where it was.*

This wasn't about weakness. This was about perception. I reached for my lenses.

Not a prescription. Not a magnification. But a prism, oriented to shift how her system mapped space. A lens that speaks not to clarity—but to integration. One that would reintroduce her to gravity. To posture. To self-location.

She put them on. And in that moment—everything changed. She stood. She paused. Her eyes widened. And then, with a mix of disbelief and joy, she dropped the cane.

*And she **waltzed**.*

Right there in my office hallway. A soft, floating rhythm emerged from her body—the kind of movement that couldn't be faked. Her spine lifted. Her head aligned. She was no longer compensating—she was expressing.

She turned to me, tears in her eyes. She didn't ask how it worked. She didn't need to. She had returned to herself.

*What's more—her brother, the skeptical ophthalmologist, would later write about our work **together**. He became a believer—not just because of the data, but because of the undeniable transformation he witnessed in his own sister.*

She is now being featured in a case series by a local hospital. But for me, the real case study happened in those few sacred seconds between stillness and motion. Between fragmentation and flow.

*When vision returned—not only to her eyes, but to her **life**.*

You've felt it before. That gut-level knowing. That moment when your body responds before your mind even catches up. It's the way your shoulders tense before a loud noise. The way your feet adjust before you consciously register uneven ground. The flutter in your stomach before you hear bad news. These aren't coincidences— they are signs of your subconscious vision at work.

You flinch before you identify the threat. You recoil from a glare before you consciously label the discomfort. You shift away from someone's gaze without knowing why. You feel the tension in a room before a word is spoken. You feel off balance in a space that's too bright, too loud, too cluttered—and you can't quite explain why.

This is vision beneath awareness. It is not imagination. It is not mysticism. It is your nervous system in action—reflexive, protective, beautifully intelligent. It is the body's first response system. The field of subconscious vision is the invisible scaffolding upon which your experience of safety, orientation, and relational presence is built.

What Is Subconscious Vision?

Subconscious vision refers to the vast array of visual processing that occurs below the level of conscious thought. It is rapid, effective, and embodied. It is vision without narrative. Vision without labels. Vision that shapes your world before you've even had a chance to name it.

This field allows you to detect danger before analysis. It allows you to sense invitation or rejection in a glance. It helps you attune to micro-expressions, posture shifts, environmental cues, and energetic presence—all without deliberate focus. It's what gives you goosebumps.

Subconscious vision does not speak in words. It speaks in orientation, tension, movement, and subtle alignment. It alters your breathing, posture, vocal tone, and somatic field long before you become "aware."

The Science Behind the Subconscious Field

Most students of optometry or any visual science are taught about the conscious visual system—from the cells in the retina to the thalamus to the visual cortex. This system is responsible for clarity, color, detail, and spatial mapping in conscious awareness.

But there's another faster, and older, visual highway: the tecto-pulvinar pathway. This route doesn't prioritize clarity. It prioritizes survival. Visual input travels from the retina to the superior colliculus, then to the pulvinar nucleus, and finally to deep structures like the amygdala and parietal cortex. This is not linear logic—it's emotional geometry. It maps how the body should respond based on prior patterns of stress, movement, and emotional memory.

The superior colliculus detects motion and shift. The pulvinar filters out noise to protect from overwhelm. The amygdala codes emotional tone before you "see" it. The parietal lobes orient the body. This system bypasses language and cognition. It is primitive, profound, and present in every moment of your life.

Vision Is a Sensory Coherence System

Subconscious vision does not operate in isolation. It collaborates and co-regulates with your vestibular system (balance), your proprioceptive system (body mapping), your auditory system (environmental awareness), and your interoceptive system (internal states).

This creates sensory coherence—a unified field of awareness where what you see, feel, hear, and sense align. When this system is working in harmony, people feel anchored, responsive, calm. When it's disrupted—through trauma, injury, overstimulation, or dysregulation—they feel scattered, reactive, or disconnected.

Sensory coherence is the nervous system's ability to say: "This moment matches what I expect. I am safe. I am oriented. I belong here." Vision is a central orchestrator of this coherence.

Emotions that Live in the Field

What we often overlook in traditional vision science—but what patients show us again and again—is that emotion lives in the visual field. Not just as expression, but as perception. Grief can tilt posture. Fear can collapse convergence. Unprocessed emotion can manifest as visual withdrawal or hypersensitivity. These aren't just metaphors. They are neurological realities—visible to the practitioner who knows how to look.

Through years of clinical work—and the development of what you will soon understand as the Neuro-Integrative Vision Model— I've come to recognize that the subconscious visual field is not only perceptual, but profoundly emotional. It stores what hasn't been spoken. It holds the residue of experience, the imprints of emotion, and—sometimes—the echoes of inheritance. It protects what once overwhelmed the system. And it carries forward what we haven't yet released.

In my one-on-one sessions, I often use a method grounded in applied kinesiology—specifically muscle testing—to access what I've come to understand as the emotional language of the visual system. This technique allows me to gently decode trapped emotional patterns that influence not just how a person sees optically, but how they orient in space, perceive safety, and engage with the world energetically.

Sometimes, these patterns trace back to early developmental experiences—like the shame a child felt being unable to read aloud in class. Other times, the emotional imprint appears to be inherited: a fear, a pressure, or a grief that did not begin with the patient but now lives within them, subtly shaping posture, orientation, and visual processing.

Here's what's most remarkable: when the emotion is witnessed, the system recalibrates. The visual field softens. Eye movements synchronize. Posture finds its natural alignment. Breathing deepens. The nervous system begins to *exhale*.

You may not always measure this shift with a Snellen chart. But you can see it in the way someone stands. You can hear it in the change in their voice. You can feel it in the space between you—something has settled.

This isn't a one-off story. It's not "alternative medicine." It's pattern recognition. And it's time we name it.

Integration with the Neuro-Integrative Model

This is why the Neuro-Integrative Vision Model cannot be reduced to acuity or even higher-order cognitive processing. It is a living model, one that recognizes that vision is a reflection of the subconscious nervous system, emotional history, and the body's attempt to organize reality in a way that feels survivable.

In some patients, I see it when a low-power lens calms their posture and breath. In others, I see it when a subconscious belief is released through somatic testing. In all of them, I see it when the body *finally feels safe enough to stop compensating*.

This work is not about mystical claims. It's about acknowledging the real, repeatable, observable changes that happen when we address vision as a whole-body, whole-history experience.

Why does this matter?

Most visual dysfunction isn't about acuity. It's about integration. We pathologize sensitivity when we should be honoring it. Children who hide from bright lights or avoid eye contact aren't being difficult—they are self-regulating. Adults who get overwhelmed in malls or under fluorescents aren't weak—they are overloaded. When you understand subconscious vision, you stop fixing the behavior and start listening to the message.

Real-World Signs of Subconscious Vision at Work

- A child cries when the lights change in a room—not because they're spoiled, but because their visual system is overstimulated.
- An adult feels "foggy" in a room with certain lighting and cannot focus.
- A patient walks straighter with a subtle lens adjustment and gets emotional—not because they understand it cognitively, but because something inside finally feels right.
- A trauma survivor panics in a crowded environment where peripheral input is chaotic.
- An athlete anticipates the play not just with skill—but with subconscious pattern recognition.

These are all signs that vision goes far beyond sight—it's deeply tied to feeling, adapting, and inner knowing. Vision is not a passive process. It doesn't reside solely in the eyes; it reflects the orientation of the entire being.

When we work with this layer of vision, we restore sensory harmony. We help people re-enter space and time with confidence. We offer more than correction—we offer regulation.

That is what the Neuro-Integrative Vision Model honors: clarity aligned with coherence, function expressed through embodiment. Your eyes are not mere cameras—they are thresholds. To body. To space. To self. To the invisible field that keeps you whole.

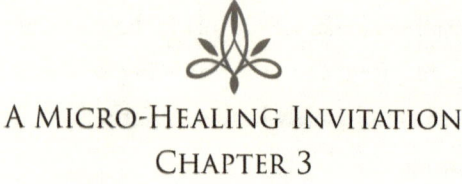

A MICRO-HEALING INVITATION
CHAPTER 3

Vision and the Subconscious

Your visual system is constantly working behind the scenes—tracking motion, filtering complexity, scanning for safety. Long before your conscious mind catches up, your eyes and nervous system have already begun to interpret the world.

This isn't mysticism—it's biology. It's also deeply personal.

Take a moment to reflect:

- Can you recall a time when your body responded before your thoughts did?

- Have you ever flinched, turned away, or felt overwhelmed—without knowing why?

Gently close your eyes. Scan your body, not for answers, but for signals.

Is there a place that feels alert? Disoriented? Heavy? Or calm?

Now, remind yourself: your subconscious visual system is designed to protect you. It's not overreacting—it's perceiving on your behalf.

What would it feel like to trust that this deeper layer of vision is not a flaw, but a form of intelligence?

Let that reframe your relationship with sensitivity.

Let it soften your expectations.

Let it remind you:

You are not broken.

You are brilliantly wired to see more than meets the eye.

4

Introducing the Neuro-Integrative Vision Model

A New Lens for Seeing Ourselves— and the World

I first met him when he was just a toddler.

He had been given the wrong dosage of medication at seven months old—an accidental overdose by the pharmacy. What followed was chaos in his nervous system. He moved constantly. His eyes didn't focus. His hearing was inconsistent. His milestones regressed. His speech was non-existent.

When he arrived at my office at twenty-two months old, his mother looked exhausted. Not from parenting—but from grief. She had lost the baby she once knew. She didn't say it out loud, but I could feel it in the way she held him. He was fading into himself, and no one could reach him.

I remember the moment I first looked into his eyes. Big. Blue. Searching.

He didn't reach for the toys I placed around him. He didn't respond to his name. He leaned forward constantly, off-balance, disconnected from gravity.

But his gaze told me everything.

This wasn't just a developmental delay. It was a collapse of **coherence**. *His body had no orientation. His brain had no map. He was adrift in space—and in himself.*

So I got to work—not to correct, but to connect. I placed a subtle yoked prism in front of his eyes—just enough to cue his body into an upright posture. I added a low-powered plus lens, one that would offer the gentlest access to focus without demand. A signal of safety.

The shift was immediate. He sat upright. His eyes twinkled. He reached for a toy—for the first time.

It was a miracle. But it wasn't magic. It was resonance. His system had been waiting for a signal that said: **You're safe. You're here**.

That moment was five years ago.

I've seen him regularly since then—changing lenses, updating prescriptions, supporting each new stage of development. We worked through spatial awareness (Body Vision), through regulation and tracking (Focus), through confidence and identity (Meaning), and even through how he relates and connects with others (Expression).

But it was his most recent visit that left me undone. He handed me a letter. Folded neatly, written in careful block letters.

His mom didn't know he'd written it.

It said:

> *Dr. Peddle,*
> *Thank you for all that you do for my eyes since I was a baby. I'm always sooo excited when I hear I'm going to see you, and every time I go to you, I'm always wondering what your MAGIC hands are going to do to my eyes.*
>
> *Love,*
> *Your favorite patient*

I teared up. Because vision therapy through lenses didn't just help him track, or focus, or balance. It helped him return to himself.

And it helped me remember that what we're really doing— through every lens, every color, every visit—is restoring connection to the inner field of knowing. The one that says:

You are not broken. You are seen. You are home.

How the Model Was Born—The Path That Chose Me

The Neuro-Integrative Vision Model wasn't something I set out to create—it was something I *began to remember*, patient by patient, moment by moment.

In my private practice, a specific kind of patient began showing up. These were children who struggled in school—not due to a lack of intelligence, but because their systems weren't integrating the way traditional models anticipated. Parents drove hours—sometimes across provinces—not for my credentials, but for the unique way I approached prescribing. My neuro-functional lens prescribing was gaining a quiet but powerful reputation. It was helping with reading speed, handwriting, copying, comprehension, even emotional regulation and confidence. And these results weren't occasional—they were consistent. But even as results spoke louder than science, I began sensing that what was happening went beyond function. There was an emotional thread, a subconscious readiness I could feel—but hadn't yet named.

Soon, something began to shift. The results I was witnessing in my patients—particularly in children struggling with reading, writing, or focus—weren't going unnoticed. Teachers started reaching out, not just to comment on a child's improvement, but to ask, with genuine curiosity, "What changed? What did you do?" Therapists began referring their clients to me after seeing transformations they couldn't quite explain. Parents began sharing their stories with other parents. Word spread.

And before I knew it, I had a waitlist that stretched six months into the future. Not because I was offering something trendy or flashy—but because something I was doing was working in a way that felt meaningful, sustainable, and deeply human. Patients weren't just seeing better. They were functioning better. They were feeling better. They were returning to themselves.

Then came the invitations—to teach, to speak, to explain how and why I was prescribing the way I was. And while I was honored, I also felt a sense of urgency. This couldn't remain the best-kept secret in optometry. It had to become something more. It had to be named, studied, taught, shared. I didn't want to be the only one seeing these results. I wanted this deeper way of seeing and supporting patients to ripple far beyond my exam room.

But when I was invited to lecture on these transformations—across Canada, the US, Europe—I realized something unsettling: **I couldn't exactly explain *why* it worked.** Not through the lens of traditional science. There were no double-blind placebo-controlled studies validating what I was seeing. There were no graphs, no charts, no consensus guidelines.

And yet, the results were undeniable.

So, I did what all seekers do when faced with something that cannot be explained: I went deeper. I dove into the neural pathways. I revisited the anatomy and physiology I had memorized years ago—but this time, I read it with new eyes. I read between the lines. I followed the threads—into the emotional brain, the limbic loops, the subconscious response systems, the somatosensory scaffolding that holds us upright *and* forms our sense of self.

And slowly, I began to see what I hadn't been taught: that vision is not just a system of sight—it is a mirror of identity. A bridge between the conscious and subconscious. A fluid, adaptive expression of a person's emotional history, genetic coding, relational blueprint, and lived experience.

There was no single study that could contain this. No controlled variable that could capture the nuance of it.

Because the truth is: every patient carries an unrepeatable matrix—a fusion of trauma, memory, perception, and resilience. And these elements don't simply influence how we feel. They shape how we see.

What was missing in our models wasn't technique. It was *interconnection*. It was the fascia of the nervous system—the web that links logic and emotion, retina and posture, movement and meaning.

The Neuro-Integrative Vision Model emerged from this understanding. A model not meant to replace science, but to *expand it*. To honor the subtle. To make room for what cannot be double-blinded but is *visibly transforming lives* every single day.

This is a model of integration. A lens that accounts for the full spectrum of human perception—from retina to resonance, from neurological processing to soul recognition.

And it begins with a question: ***What if the way you see is the way you live?***

I didn't understand the full anatomy of what was happening at the time. But I *felt* it. I've felt it thousands of times.

But one case changed everything for me. It anchored the possibility that the visual system isn't just a receiver of light—it's a messenger of readiness, of belonging, of return.

Here's that story.

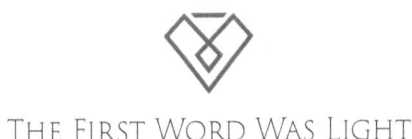

The First Word Was Light

He had never spoken a word.

Not a single one.

Four years old. Diagnosed on the autism spectrum.

Bright eyes. Quick movements. But silent.

His mother sat across from me with that kind of exhaustion only parents of non-verbal children know. A strange mix of fierce love and quiet heartbreak.

She had tried everything—speech therapy, occupational therapy, sensory integration, special diets. Every therapy with every acronym.

And now, she was here. Not expecting much. Just hoping for some visual support.

But when I looked at him—really looked—I could feel it.

*His system wasn't shut down. It was **guarded.***

His eyes flickered, scanning constantly. His breath was high in his chest. His nervous system wasn't in language mode. It was in survival.

*I knew he didn't need just vision support—he needed a **shift.** Something that would cue his system that it was safe to let go.*

I added the subtlest tint to his lenses—one designed to stimulate the parasympathetic nervous system.

Not to "calm him down" but to invite him in.

And the moment he put them on . . . He turned to his mother. Looked her straight in the eye.

And said,

"Mom."

Just that.

But it wasn't just a word. It was a portal. A rupture in silence. A return. A miracle.

His mother gasped—covering her mouth, tears streaming.

My throat caught. We just sat there, time dissolving.

She reached for his hand, and he didn't pull away. He looked again.

And this time, he smiled.

*Since that day, I've never seen color the same way. Because that tint didn't just change his visual input—It changed his **access**.*

It showed me, again, that vision is not about clarity. It's about connection. That moment wasn't the result of a lens alone. It was the nervous system saying yes—to presence, to relationship, to the unseen signal that said: you are safe to emerge.

He didn't need coaxing or drilling or flashcards. He needed **resonance**.

And in that moment, A child who had never spoken said the most sacred word a mother can hear—

Not because he was taught to. But because his system finally said, **"Now. It's safe. Speak."**

And I swear to you—he knew I saw him. Not just his prescription. Not just his nervous system.

Him.

Because that's the thing about children—especially the non-verbal ones. They know. They read us. Long before we speak.

Long before we ask a question.

*And often—***they read me as clearly as I read them.***

I've had sessions where I can **feel** *what a child needs before they look at the eye chart. Where I know which lens to pull, which color to use—because their body and energy already told me.*

And when I hold that energy field with stillness and trust, I've watched them meet me there. It's not something I was taught. It's not in the textbooks.

But it's real.

There's a kind of telepathy that happens when you meet a nervous system in safety.

A non-verbal language between souls. It's the space where the real healing happens.

That little boy didn't just say "Mom" that day.

*He said: **I trust you. I'm ready to come forward.***

And in that moment, I felt it in my entire body. The sacred agreement:

"I see you. I believe in you. I won't rush you. But I'll never stop holding the space for you to rise."

It wasn't about clarity. It wasn't about acuity. It was about resonance.

And that is the essence of the Integrative Field—this fifth "circle" that lives beneath every transformation.

It's time to name it.

The Next Model

By now, you've seen how the Classical Structural Model taught us about anatomy and ocular health. How the Visual Functional Model expanded into movement and development. How the Neuro-Cognitive Model brought in attention, processing, and brain function.

But none of them accounted for what clinicians feel in the room—the moment a lens makes someone cry, or a posture shifts before words are spoken.

They couldn't explain why a trauma survivor feels more stable in space before their brain can articulate why. Or why a child with autism makes eye contact for the first time with a gentle tint in place.

These were not outliers. They were evidence.

We needed a model that:

- Includes subconscious and embodied perception
- Recognizes the emotional and intuitive tone of vision
- Honors the nervous system's need for safety and resonance
- Connects visual processing to identity, memory, expression, and healing

The Neuro-Integrative Vision Model does not discard the past—it completes it. It builds on everything we've learned, and brings forward everything we've felt but couldn't name.

How the Model Was Discovered

This model then unfolded over years. Not through academic study alone, but through presence.

Through real human moments:

- A child bursting into tears with a new lens—before any verbal description
- A patient saying, "I feel like I can breathe again," after a microprism shift
- A parent whispering, "This is the first time I've seen my child look back"

Unknowing to me, it started during my residency, my lectures, my hands-on sessions. Through the stories patients told with their eyes, their posture, their breath.

And underneath it all was a longing: to create a model that honored the science and the sacred. A model where the nervous system and soul could both be seen.

This model was revealed—not invented.

The Five Fields of Vision

Unlike the Classical Structural Model or even Skeffington's Four Circles—which were widely taught and passed down through generations of optometrists—the **fields** within the Neuro-Integrative Vision Model are not inherited frameworks. They're not borrowed from textbooks or clinical traditions, but they are based on our previous scaffolds. They are named. Intentionally. They arose from years of clinical pattern recognition, deep listening, and immersion in the subtle, often unspoken language of the nervous system. These fields are a way of organizing the vast, layered experience of vision—not only as a mechanical function or a skill set, but as a dynamic, integrative process that bridges the body, the brain, and the subconscious self. They also reflect the way the nervous system speaks—through patterns, not parts. Through resonance, not just reaction.

This language didn't come from outside of me. It came through me—built from both science and soul, clinical precision and intuitive knowing. And though the fields are not yet found in formal curricula, they represent what many practitioners have long sensed but struggled to name. Now, we name them. Together.

The Neuro-Integrative Vision Model organizes vision into five interrelated fields. These are based on previous models that have shaped my clinical skills. These are not silos. They are dynamic, flowing currents. Each field represents a way the visual system interacts with the body, the brain, the world—and the self.

1. The Field of Body Vision

This is the most primal layer of vision—the sense of where you are in space, and whether that space feels safe. It is shaped by the integration of the visual, vestibular, and proprioceptive systems. It includes midline awareness, balance, postural tone, and spatial mapping.

Patients with disturbances in this field may feel disoriented, dizzy, clumsy, or "out of body." Children may walk on their toes, lean forward, or avoid movement. Adults may bump into doorways or feel ungrounded in crowds.

This field governs your embodied orientation in the world. And when it is regulated—everything else begins to settle.

2. The Field of Focus

This field involves the regulation of visual input. It includes convergence, divergence, tracking, saccades, visual attention, and filtering. But beyond mechanics, it reflects how the nervous system chooses what to engage—and what to let go. In the Neuro-Integrative Vision Model, focus is not about eyesight—it's about insight. It's how the system chooses where to place its attention and where to let go.

Children with dysregulation in this field may struggle to attend, fatigue quickly, or become overwhelmed in busy environments. Adults may describe fogginess, "eye strain," or visual chaos.

This field is deeply linked to the autonomic nervous system. Visual overfocus can reflect sympathetic overdrive. Avoidance can reflect dorsal shutdown.

Focus is not a skill—it's a state. And it must feel safe to be engaged.

3. The Field of Meaning

This is the interpretive field—the space where recognition, identification, and memory meet.

It includes object and face recognition (ventral stream), pattern recognition, visual memory, and symbolic understanding. It is tied to culture, belief systems, trauma, and narrative.

This is where the brain assigns story to what is seen. A face becomes "friend" or "threat." A word becomes "confusing" or "empowering."

When dysregulated, this field can contribute to identity fragmentation, mislabeling, or visual triggers rooted in past trauma.

It's not just what you see—it's what it means to you.

4. The Field of Expression

This is the field of relational vision. It includes eye contact, gaze regulation, emotional communication through the eyes, and the visual feedback loop that supports co-regulation.

This field links to the social nervous system (polyvagal theory), facial expression, speech, and gesture.

Children who avoid eye contact or adults who feel "not seen" often carry dysregulation here. Some overcompensate—holding intense eye contact as a form of control. Others collapse or dissociate.

This is where vision becomes a mirror. It's where we are seen—and where we learn to see ourselves.

5. The Field of Inner Vision

This is the most subtle and most powerful field.

It includes blindsight, intuition, energetic perception, and subconscious visual processing through the tecto-pulvinar system. It also includes the limbic system—the emotional filter that shapes perception before thought.

This is the field that senses before it sees. The one that flinches before the object is identified. The one that knows.

This field has been dismissed by traditional science—but it lives in every practitioner who has ever said: "I just had a feeling this would work."

It is the field of soul-sight. The place where resonance guides the hand.

While each field offers a doorway, it's often Inner Vision that holds the key to unlocking transformation—the place where healing begins before words are found.

A Model of Interconnection, Not Hierarchy

These five fields are not steps. They are interwoven.

A trauma in the Field of Body Vision can create avoidance in Focus. A collapse in Expression can dull Inner Vision. A rigid lens in Meaning can limit how safely one engages with Body Vision.

Healing is not about fixing one field—it's about re-establishing coherence among them.

That's what this model does.

What This Changes

The Neuro-Integrative Vision Model changes how we practice, how we teach, and how we see each other. It gives clinicians language for the ineffable. It validates the intuitive hits we've always felt. It shows patients that their symptoms are not only real—but meaningful. It invites the public to see vision as a system of regulation, relationship, and remembrance. It is not just a map of perception.

It is a guide for returning to the self. This is the Neuro-Integrative Vision Model.

The next lens. The deeper truth. The beginning of real vision.

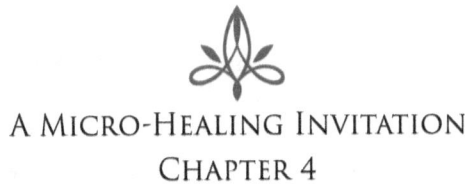

A Micro-Healing Invitation
Chapter 4

Introducing the Neuro-Integrative Vision Model

You've just been introduced to a model that reframes vision as more than sight—as a reflection of how we sense, interpret, and move through the world. The Neuro-Integrative Vision Model isn't just about the eyes. It's about coherence. It's about connection.

Take a quiet moment to pause and ask:

What if your visual system has been telling your story all along?

What if your posture, your sensitivity, and your reactions to space are not isolated symptoms—but expressions of how your system has learned to see and survive?

Let yourself trace this idea gently:

Where have you been trying to "fix" something that might actually be part of a deeper pattern?

Could the way you engage with the world—your clarity, fatigue, even your movement—be part of your vision speaking?

This model doesn't offer formulas.

It offers integration.

It gives language to what your system has known all along.

Let yourself feel the possibility of coherence—not as something to strive for, but something already within reach.

Because when vision becomes integrative, healing stops being about correction . . .

And becomes a return to wholeness.

ADDED NOTE: Science Behind the Intuition: The Brain Pathways That "See" Without Words

Although many think of vision as a conscious process driven by the visual cortex, the truth is—some of our deepest visual awareness bypasses conscious sight entirely.

One of the most important pathways involved in this subconscious visual processing is the tecto–pulvinar–amygdala pathway.

- This circuit routes visual information from the superior colliculus (part of the midbrain's tectum) to the pulvinar nucleus of the thalamus, and then directly into the amygdala—the emotional center of the brain.
- It's fast. It's non-verbal.
- And it's deeply emotional and intuitive.

This is the same system active in *blindsight* patients—individuals who are cortically blind, yet still respond to visual stimuli without conscious awareness.

In intuitive clinical encounters—especially with sensitive or non-verbal individuals—this system is often in full activation.

The practitioner and the patient may be exchanging visual-emotional information *beneath conscious awareness*, reading each other through body language, energy shifts, facial micro-expressions, and light-induced nervous system cues.

In my work, this isn't just theory—it's felt experience. It's the field I operate in. And for my patients—especially those who don't respond to linear treatment—this is where true healing begins.

5

THE FIELD OF BODY VISION

Before We See, We Land: The Sensory Field That Says, "You Are Safe"

I've lost count of the number of times I've heard some version of:

"That's too low to make a difference."

"That prism is basically nothing."

"Why would you prescribe that? It's not even a full diopter."

There's a belief in our profession—and in many fields—that only what's measurable is meaningful. That if you can't chart a change on paper, you can't call it progress.

But then there are the moments that crack that idea wide open.

Like the patient who couldn't enter a grocery store because of visual overwhelm . . . until I added 0.50 base-in prism over one eye, and they stopped clenching their jaw for the first time in years.

Or the child with chronic tantrums and poor balance, whose emotional regulation improved *within a week* after a +0.25 lens shift brought their nervous system back into a range where they could simply feel safe.

The numbers were small. The changes? Massive.

The truth is, these microlenses and microprisms are **tuning forks** for the nervous system. They don't shout. They whisper. And when the body is ready, it listens.

But what's almost harder than getting the prescription right . . . is *trusting it*. Especially when the shift we're inviting isn't only optical—it's neurological. It's energetic. It's the subtle moment when the body says "yes" to a new map.

Trusting the prescription is so difficult because we've been taught to justify every choice. To predict every outcome. To write down a diagnosis code that satisfies someone else's need for certainty. So when I started leaning into this quiet form of prescribing—this way of feeling the system instead of forcing it—I had to push through a thick fog of guilt.

Was I doing this for the patient . . . or for me? Would my college approve? Would my peers judge me? Would someone assume I was trying to sell glasses that weren't "necessary"?

But I couldn't unsee what I had seen. And I couldn't unknow what I now knew:

These "insignificant" lenses were changing people's lives.

Not because of what they corrected. But because of what they *opened*. They didn't just align vision—they reoriented perception. They tuned the nervous system toward safety. And often, they did something even more profound: they helped the system remember itself.

That's the thing about working with vision as an energetic and functional system—it doesn't always follow the rules of optics. It follows the truth of the body. Of the moment.

And when we trust that . . .

The tiniest lens can become the doorway to a completely new reality.

Practitioner's Reflection: Prescribing Small, Seeing Big

If you've ever hesitated to prescribe a low plus or subtle prism because it "wasn't enough"—or because you feared judgment from your college or peers—this reflection is for you.

You are not alone.

Many of us have been trained to fear our own instincts. To trust numbers over nervous systems. To feel guilty when what we feel isn't backed by what we were taught to measure. But your perception is your power. And the nervous system doesn't wait for permission to shift. It knows what it needs. Vision is not always a system waiting to be corrected. Sometimes, it's a system waiting to be acknowledged. And when we prescribe from that place—with presence, not pressure—something ancient and wise comes forward. Every time you honor a subtle prescription, you are not just helping a patient—you are shifting the paradigm. You are saying: I trust what I see. I trust what I feel. I trust the intelligence of this system. So prescribe gently. Boldly. Reverently. The lens doesn't have to be big to be sacred.

Before we ever name an object, before we learn to read, write, or engage in the complex coordination of focus and eye contact, our visual system is busy asking one foundational question: "Am I safe here?" But the response to that question doesn't arise in words. It isn't processed through logic or even cognition. It is answered through the body— through shifts in posture, subtle adjustments in orientation, and the gut-level sense of whether the environment is known, unknown, stable, or threatening.

For more information about prisms and low-powered lenses, please see the Appendix B, found on page 159.

This bodily perception, this felt experience of being "in space," is what I call the Field of Body Vision. It is the root system beneath all other aspects of vision. It is what enables a child to feel grounded enough to sit still. What allows an adult to walk confidently into a room. What informs posture, movement, spatial orientation, and ultimately, the ability to remain present in one's own body.

Not every healing story has a dramatic before-and-after. Some unfold quietly, over weeks, asking only for trust. But then comes a moment—unexpected, beautiful, undeniable—when the healing is felt. When the system says, *I'm ready.*

This was one of those moments.

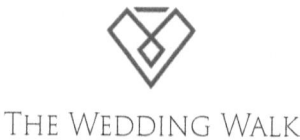

THE WEDDING WALK

She came into my office not calmly—but shaken.

Tears welled in her eyes as she stood in the doorway, her body tense, her words trembling.

*"I don't know if you can help me," she said, "but I saw the words **vision therapy** on your sign, and I thought . . . maybe this is my last shot."*

She was twenty-nine years old. A year earlier, she'd been in a "minor" motor vehicle accident. Since then, her world had been spinning—literally. She had tried everything: vestibular therapy, physiotherapy, chiropractic, craniosacral, neuro consults, nutritional support. Nothing worked. Movement overwhelmed her. Crowds triggered her. She couldn't go to busy spaces, drive comfortably, or tolerate even moderate visual stimulation.

And in six months . . . she was getting married.

"I don't think I'll be able to walk down the aisle without falling or looking like I'm drunk," she said, holding her breath. "I'm terrified that on my wedding day, I'll be dizzy and overwhelmed. I don't want to feel like this. Not then."

She was skeptical, but underneath that skepticism, I felt it: **surrender**. *She wasn't here to debate. She was here because something inside her* **wanted** *to believe there was still a path forward.*

I booked her in for a comprehensive exam and began working with the delicate balance between urgency and trust. She had a timeline. A clock ticking in her nervous system. But I knew this work doesn't respond well to pressure. The more we push, the more the nervous system resists.

She needed to get better, yes—but more than that, she needed to feel safe.

So I explained this to her. Gently, but clearly. "This isn't a quick fix," I said. "But we can walk slowly, and we can walk steadily. If we follow your system instead of forcing it, you **will** *get there."*

She agreed. And something in her softened. We began vision therapy—twenty sessions over the months that followed. I watched her learn to stabilize her gaze again. We rebuilt her visual midline, integrated her tracking and vestibular input, and slowly reintroduced movement tolerance.

Bit by bit, she came back into herself.

And then—during her final session before the wedding—she walked across the room with ease.

She turned. Smiled. Spun in place. No dizziness. No fear. She stood tall and steady and said, "I can't believe it . . . I feel like **me** *again."*

The following month she handed me a thank-you note with a photo—her in her wedding dress. Radiant. Grounded. Present.

"You were part of my day," she said. "Not just because I could walk . . . but because I could be **there**. *Fully."*

Vision therapy has the power to do more than enhance visual acuity—it can reawaken a person's sense of being. Beyond symptom reduction, it fosters presence and integration. We didn't just improve her eyesight; we synchronized her entire system. That coherence is the foundation of meaningful healing.

The system doesn't want to be rushed.

It wants to be listened to.

And when we do . . . **miracles happen right on time.**

What Is Body Vision?

Body Vision refers to the deeply interconnected relationship between the visual system and our bodily sense of space, balance, and motion. It is not about clarity or acuity. It's about knowing where your body ends and where the environment begins. It is a form of embodied orientation that arises from visual-spatial cues and is processed pre-cognitively.

This field of perception integrates several major sensory systems:

- Proprioception: the internal mapping of body position and movement
- Vestibular function: which orients the body to gravity, motion, and balance
- Motor coordination: the ability to walk, reach, balance, and stabilize

It is through Body Vision that you can instinctively walk through a doorway without bumping into the frame, navigate a staircase without consciously calculating each step, or sense that something is "off" in a space even if everything appears normal.

When this system is working, the world feels reliable. The body feels aligned. There is a quiet sense of coherence between inner and outer environments. When it's not working, however, the nervous system is constantly compensating, and that effort becomes emotionally and physically exhausting.

Signs of Body Vision Dysfunction

When Body Vision is dysregulated, the symptoms may appear behavioral, emotional, or cognitive—but they are deeply rooted in the somatic nervous system. People may appear clumsy, anxious, resistant to movement, or hypersensitive to open spaces. Children may toe-walk, slouch, avoid eye contact, or seem unable to sit still—not because they are inattentive, but because their bodies are unsure of where they are.

Common signs include:

- Clumsiness or poor motor timing
- Difficulty walking in straight lines or turning corners without disorientation
- Discomfort in wide open or visually chaotic environments
- Poor posture, leaning, or rigidity
- A tendency to avoid movement or physical play
- Unexplained anxiety, especially in unfamiliar settings

These signs often go misunderstood or misdiagnosed when, in fact, they may stem from a lack of trust in the spatial field—a body that doesn't fully believe it is safe to move.

The Neurology of Body Vision

The Field of Body Vision is primarily mediated by the magnocellular visual pathways, which specialize in detecting motion, depth, and spatial orientation. These pathways operate faster than the parvocellular system (responsible for detail and color) and are more directly tied to subconscious movement and survival behaviors.

The tecto-pulvinar pathway—an ancient visual route—also plays a central role here. Input from the retina travels to the superior colliculus, which reflexively detects motion and helps orient the body toward or away from stimuli. From there, signals pass through the pulvinar nucleus, which filters and prioritizes what sensory information is forwarded for further processing.

This entire system is intimately connected with:

- The vestibular nuclei, which govern balance and gravitational orientation
- The cerebellum, responsible for motor coordination and timing
- The parietal lobes, which construct spatial maps of the environment and body
- The spinal postural reflexes, which adjust stance and muscle tone in real time

In other words, Body Vision is not "just" visual. It is an integrated, multisensory field of perception that regulates posture, emotion, and readiness for interaction. It is also one of the most subconscious. It's where blindsight, reflexes, and inherited spatial maps quietly shape our reality—long before thought arrives. This is why healing often begins here: not in the eyes, but in the felt sense of belonging in one's own body.

Why This Field Matters

Too often, we focus on visual skills like tracking, focusing, or reading without asking the foundational questions: "Does this person feel safe in space? Do they know where they are in relation to their environment?"

No cognitive or therapeutic intervention can fully take root if the nervous system does not feel anchored. If the brain is unsure whether the body is safe in the environment, all higher-level processing—attention, memory, learning—will be impaired.

We must begin with body-first healing. Because the body is the first lens. It tells us whether the environment is safe, whether space can be trusted, and whether presence is possible.

The Day the World Became Real Again

She was a woman in her early thirties. Six months prior, she had been in what doctors described as an insignificant car accident. No visible injuries. No fractures. Nothing requiring hospitalization. And yet, her life hadn't felt the same since.

She couldn't walk a straight line. She felt foggy and disoriented in crowded places. She described herself as feeling "not fully in the room." A supermarket would send her into a full-body spiral—overwhelmed by lights, motion, and visual input she couldn't process.

She had seen multiple professionals—physiotherapists, neurologists, vestibular specialists—but still, no answers.

When she arrived at my office, she looked exhausted. She was holding back tears before the exam even began. "I know this sounds strange," she said, "but I feel like my body doesn't trust where it is."

And I knew exactly what she meant.

Her Fakuda stepping test was the clearest marker: with eyes closed, she rotated significantly to the left. Her nervous system was unable to maintain alignment in space without visual anchors. Her body wasn't grounded.

I prescribed a pair of yoked prisms—very subtle. Just enough to shift her midline and vertical orientation.

She walked the hallway once, paused, and turned back slowly. Her hand went to her chest.

"It feels like I'm back in my body again," she whispered. It wasn't just about posture. We gave her back her grounding. Her presence.

Her place in the world.

Body Vision Is a Pathway to Safety

When you support the Field of Body Vision, you are not merely improving physical function. You are nurturing the nervous system's sense of safety. You are helping a person feel more real, more embodied, more capable of existing in the world without fear of misalignment or collapse.

Body Vision is the beginning of integration. It is the sensory groundwork for regulation, perception, and emotional resilience. When this field is activated and restored, healing is no longer just possible—it becomes inevitable.

In the Neuro-Integrative Vision Model, Body Vision is not a step—it's a gateway. It's the first reconnection point between the nervous system and the self. And when we meet it with reverence, the rest begins to unfold.

A MICRO-HEALING INVITATION
CHAPTER 5

The Body Field: Perceiving Safety, Space, and Self
Before we can focus, engage, or assign meaning, the body needs one essential signal: *you are safe here.*

This chapter invited you to explore the Field of Body Vision—the foundation of all perception. This field isn't about clarity or control. It's about orientation. It's about whether your system knows where you are in space, and whether that space feels safe.

Take a slow, steady breath.

Then ask yourself:

- **Do I feel grounded in my body—or often just slightly outside of it?**

- Do I move through space with trust, or with quiet tension I've learned to ignore?

There's no right answer—only awareness.

When the Field of Body Vision is dysregulated, we often focus on the symptoms: restlessness, poor posture, avoidance of movement. But the body isn't malfunctioning. It's adapting. It's doing its best to find stability in a world that doesn't always feel safe.

Today, try this:

Take a walk. Gently. Slowly. Let your feet truly meet the ground.

Notice how your gaze responds when your body softens into gravity.

Don't correct. Don't perform. Just notice.

Your body doesn't need perfection to feel safe.

It needs presence. It needs your permission to return.

6

THE FIELD OF FOCUS

The Inner Compass of Attention, Intention, and Meaning

Once the body has anchored itself in space—once a sense of safety and orientation has been established—another essential function of the visual system comes online: the ability to select. To prioritize. To direct attention toward what matters most and filter out what doesn't. In this model, focus does not refer to optical clarity or accommodation—it refers to the nervous system's capacity to attend, filter, and sustain engagement with meaning. Focus is not simply an academic tool—it is a survival strategy, shaped by lived experience. And for many patients, that strategy has become reflexive, protective, and exhausted. In a world overflowing with visual stimuli, this capacity is not just a luxury—it is fundamental to regulation, learning, and human connection.

This is the Field of Focus. It is the space where vision becomes more than perception—it becomes intention. This field governs how the nervous system sifts through sensory information to decide: "What should I look at? What should I ignore? Where should I place my awareness right now?"

And just as the Field of Body Vision roots us in presence, the Field of Focus allows us to sustain it. To direct our gaze. To maintain attention. To track meaning. It is not simply about seeing clearly—it is about seeing meaningfully because vision doesn't just perceive. It chooses. And that choice lives in the body before it ever reaches the mind.

What Is Focus in the Visual System?

In the Neuro-Integrative Model, focus is not about eyesight—it's about insight. It's how the system chooses where to place its attention and where to let go.

Focus in the visual context goes far beyond the optical clarity measured by a letter chart. True visual focus involves a symphony of skills that enable sustained, selective, and adaptive attention. It includes:

- Convergence and divergence: the eyes' ability to team effectively across distances
- Smooth pursuits and saccades: tracking objects in motion and jumping across text or scenes
- Visual attention: selecting relevant stimuli amidst noise
- Inhibition: blocking out unnecessary or conflicting input
- Visual-motor integration: coordinating vision with body movements

These skills, while often taught as mechanics, are deeply shaped by emotional tone and nervous system readiness. Focus, at its core, is a state of safety.

This domain of vision is crucial for academic tasks like reading, copying, and writing—but it also affects emotional regulation, social interaction, and even breath control. When the Field of Focus is functioning well, individuals can shift attention with ease, stay engaged without fatigue, and recover from distraction without distress.

When it is dysregulated, however, the impact is profound. The person may appear inattentive or hyper-focused, overwhelmed or shut down. Their system is not broken—it is simply overloaded.

The Neurology of Focus

The Field of Focus draws upon an intricate network of cortical and subcortical structures that guide attention, regulate arousal, and manage gaze. Key areas include:

- The parietal lobe, which helps sustain attention and process spatial context
- The frontal eye fields, located in the prefrontal cortex, which are responsible for voluntary gaze shifts, goal setting, and executive planning of eye movements
- The superior colliculus, which governs reflexive eye movements and fast shifts in attention to novel or threatening stimuli
- The reticular activating system (RAS), a brainstem network involved in arousal, alertness, and the transition between attention and rest
- The dorsal stream, also known as the "where" pathway, which helps locate objects in space and guides motor coordination.

The Field of Focus is also modulated by the sympathetic nervous system, particularly in moments of threat or overstimulation. In these states, attention narrows. Visual fields constrict. The nervous system retreats from exploration and shifts into protection. This is why many patients don't struggle with focus because of a deficit—but because their system has learned that vigilance is safer than engagement. We cannot talk about focus without acknowledging fear. They are neurologically intertwined.

Why Focus Breaks Down

This system is exquisitely sensitive. Even minor disruptions in posture, lighting, visual teaming, or emotional regulation can overwhelm the capacity to focus.

Common stressors that compromise the Field of Focus include:

- Visual clutter or environmental overstimulation
- Unstable binocular vision or convergence insufficiency
- Flickering lights or screens
- Emotional overload or trauma history
- Vestibular or proprioceptive disorientation

When these factors are present, the nervous system may prioritize survival over attention. A child who appears "distracted" may, in fact, be flooded. An adult who "can't focus" may be defending against a sea of visual and emotional input. This is not a failure of will—it is a brilliant, protective adaptation. And when we view it through a neuro-integrative lens, we see that what looks like distraction is often a language of overwhelm—a system saying, "I'm trying to stay safe."

The Boy Who Finally Found the Line

He was nine years old, bright, and creative, but falling behind. His teachers described him as distracted. His parents were told it was ADHD. He had tried medication, but it hadn't helped. Reading was a daily battle. He described the words as "jumping" off the page, and he often gave up after a few minutes—frustrated, tearful, defeated.

When I evaluated him, I saw something different. His convergence was weak, especially under stress. His saccades were inconsistent, his eyes losing their place after each line. He wasn't lazy—he was visually overloaded.

I prescribed a low-powered base-down prism and a gentle plus lens to reduce visual demand. I didn't explain what it would do. I just handed him a book.

He opened it. Sat still. Began to read—out loud. No skipping. No rubbing his eyes. No sighing.

After a minute, he looked up. "I can follow the words now," he said. His father, seemingly skeptical at first, was now stunned.

*But what changed wasn't just his reading. His whole system softened. His posture changed. His breathing slowed. He didn't just find the line on the page—**he found the line within himself**. A line between survival and presence. Between effort* *and trust. He wasn't fighting his body anymore. He wasn't trying to survive the page. He was present.*

That is the power of the Field of Focus.

Focus and the Subconscious Field

Focus is not only a conscious act. Long before a person voluntarily attends to something, their subconscious mind has already begun filtering the world. The tecto-pulvinar pathway—along with other subconscious systems—sorts through stimuli and categorizes them as relevant, irrelevant, or threatening. This pre-conscious filtering determines what rises into awareness and what is dismissed. In the Neuro-Integrative Vision Model, this is where we meet the hidden drivers of perception—those emotional, inherited, or energetic imprints that live beneath the threshold of thought.

When this system is shaped by trauma, neurodivergence, or sensory imbalance, a person may become hyper-vigilant, shut down, or stuck in patterns of visual defense. The world can feel like too much, and attention becomes not just difficult—but painful.

This is why the Field of Focus must be addressed with both scientific precision and compassionate understanding. We are not simply training attention—we are restoring a person's relationship with space, sensation, and self. A lens may reduce convergence demand—but what it's really doing is creating enough space for the system to stop bracing.

The Gift of Focus Work

When we intervene in this field with subtle lenses, prisms, or environmental support, the results are often profound. Children begin to enjoy learning again. Adults report clarity in spaces that once overwhelmed them. Teachers notice improved behavior. Parents notice emotional shifts.

We are not just changing how people see—we are changing how they *engage*.

Because when a person can choose where to place their attention, they reclaim agency. They begin to feel capable, confident, and curious. The world feels less chaotic. And beneath the clinical outcomes lies something even more powerful: a shift in relationship. With space. With stillness. With the self. And the self—once fragmented—feels whole again.

Focus is not only academic. It is emotional. Energetic. Transformational. Because when the Field of Focus returns, we don't just pay attention—we connect. Focus doesn't return because we force it—it returns because we restore the conditions for safety. And from there, attention becomes not a task, but a choice.

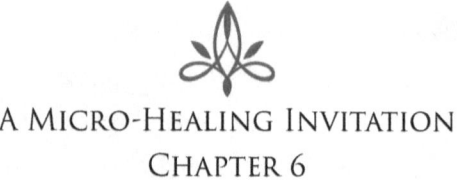

A Micro-Healing Invitation
Chapter 6

The Field of Focus: Filtering, Attending, and Regulating

Once the body feels stable in space, the visual system begins to ask a quieter, more complex question: **What deserves my attention right now?**

The Field of Focus isn't about willpower. It's about capacity.

It's the brain's ability to tune in, to filter out, and to hold steady—without overload.

When this field is regulated, your world feels manageable. When it's dysregulated, everything competes for attention—and the system becomes fatigued.

Take a moment to reflect:

- Do you often feel overstimulated by movement, brightness, or cluttered environments?

- Do you struggle to stay engaged—or hyper-focus to the point of exhaustion?

These are not personality traits.

They are **neuro-visual cues**—your system's way of maintaining regulation in a world that doesn't always allow it.

Here's a simple practice to support recalibration:

Find one object nearby.

Let your eyes land on it—not as a task, but as an anchor.

Notice your breath.

Notice if your body starts to settle.

You're not training attention.

You're giving your system permission to *rest* in it.

Sometimes, the clearest vision comes not from effort—but from simplicity.

7

THE FIELD OF MEANING

The Stories We See and the Beliefs that Shape Us

THE DOCTOR WHO FOUND HER VOICE

She was a brilliant optometrist—highly trained, respected, analytical.

*She had come to one of my prescribing workshops, the kind where we let go of all the textbook rules and just **feel** what a lens does to the system. I had paired everyone up and asked them to imagine they were six years old again—curious, playful, and unafraid to explore. I wanted them to throw away all preconceived notions of lenses, optics, refraction, and power. I wanted them to feel* *safe—to be vulnerable, like an innocent child playing with a treasure box of lenses.*

*The doctor I'm thinking of was paired with another practitioner. They began testing lenses on each other, the way I had demonstrated. When her partner placed a very low-powered lens in front of her eyes—barely measurable in prescription strength—she **threw it off instantly**.*

"I can't wear that," she said. "I feel like I can't speak."

The room went silent. I gently asked, "When did you feel like you lost your voice?"

She paused. Her eyes welled up. "When I first got glasses," she said. "I was six."

*The words hung in the air, reverberating with memory. Her body knew. Her system had stored that moment— as a visual prescription, and as a story of self. A story that said: **When you wear glasses, you are not heard. You are not yourself.***

That moment became a turning point for her. Over the weeks that followed, she wrote to me and shared that the emotion she uncovered that day was anger. Not just about the glasses—but about feeling silenced, unseen, misunderstood.

She began working with that emotion. Reframing the meaning she had internalized. And in doing so, her prescribing style shifted too. But more than that—she shifted.

*She stopped "fixing vision" and started **understanding vision**.*

Seeing the story behind the eyes. Holding space for the nervous system to rewrite the narrative.

She didn't just find a lens that day. She found her voice. And what changed wasn't just her prescription—it was her perceptual identity. Her relationship to what she saw, and what it meant, shifted. And that shift lives in the Field of Meaning.

Once the body feels anchored in space, and the nervous system is able to direct attention without being overwhelmed, a new layer of visual processing begins to unfold—one that reaches beyond posture and presence. This is the layer of interpretation. It is where vision moves from input to insight, from sensory to symbolic. At this stage, the visual system begins to ask more complex questions: "What does this mean?" "What am I looking at?" "And what does it say about me?"

This is the Field of Meaning—the dimension of visual processing where story, belief, and emotion are woven into perception. It is the lens through which we attach significance to what we see. In the Neuro-Integrative Vision Model, this is where vision becomes entangled with story—and where healing must meet both the image and the imprint. Whether consciously or not, we are always assigning meaning to our environment, to other people's faces, to text on a page, and to our own reflections. These interpretations are shaped not only by cognition but by memory, emotional experience, and deeply embedded subconscious associations.

Meaning-making is not a deliberate act. It is automatic. And because it happens below awareness, it often escapes the scope of traditional assessment. This is why so many visual-emotional wounds go unspoken—and why they must be witnessed with both science and stillness. And because it's automatic, it is also powerful—capable of reinforcing identity, triggering trauma, or shaping a lifetime of beliefs.

Vision as a Storytelling System

Every time we encounter a visual stimulus—whether a person, object, or word—our brain doesn't simply catalog its size, shape, or color. Instead, it compares that input to a vast archive of stored experiences, memories, and emotional contexts. It references the past to interpret the present. Meaning is a survival filter. It's how the nervous system says: 'This is safe. This is not. This is who I am here. It fills in gaps with assumptions, beliefs, and emotional tone.

This internal storytelling process is not inherently conscious. Two individuals can look at the same face and perceive entirely different realities—one might feel warmth and connection, while another senses judgment or threat. The object has not changed, but the lens through which it is perceived has.

These stories—crafted by the Field of Meaning—are deeply personal. In my work with the subconscious field, I've seen these meanings etched not just into cognition but into the body—into breath patterns, postural cues, eye muscle tone, and emotional reflexes. They are constructed from countless visual encounters, many of which occurred before the brain had the language to explain them. Early facial expressions from caregivers, the quality of eye contact during moments of distress, the emotional tone of school environments—all of these are imprinted into the visual-emotional map.

What Shapes the Field of Meaning?

The Field of Meaning is not hardwired. It is built. Layered. Molded through repeated exposure, emotional tone, and contextual associations. Influential factors include:

- Cultural norms and language frameworks
- Early childhood interactions and facial mirroring
- Family dynamics and patterns of eye contact
- Implicit and explicit bias
- Emotional trauma or chronic stress
- School environments and learning-based experiences
- Societal beauty standards and visual representations of identity

A child who is consistently scolded when making eye contact may begin to associate direct gaze with shame or conflict. Conversely, a child who receives calm, attuned visual connection may build associations of safety and love. These micro-moments create meaning templates, which then influence how visual input is interpreted for years—if not decades.

When the World Turned
Black and White

I had been seeing him for years. A sweet boy—gentle, quiet, and lost in a way that tugged at your heart. He was one of three—triplets. Two girls and one boy, all of whom had been in a car accident when they were just two and a half years old.

After the accident, his sisters bounced back with some therapy. Occupational and physical support got them moving forward again. They thrived in school, adjusted well socially, and resumed life with relatively few long-term issues. But him? His mother told me, "He changed." And I could see it.

He had become quiet, withdrawn. Something about him had retreated deep inward. His balance was terrible—he was always falling. He couldn't run in a straight line. Riding a bike was out of the question. We tried everything—prisms, plus lenses, vision therapy, nervous system work—layered carefully, compassionately, over the years.

But he didn't respond.

And it wasn't because he wasn't trying. He just . . . couldn't click. There was no moment of awakening, no breakthrough. Just years of gentle effort met with blankness. Still, I stayed with him. We all did.

Then one day—he was eleven by now—he came into my office and said, quietly:

"Sometimes at school . . . everything turns black and white."

*It wasn't a metaphor. He meant it **literally**.*

As a practitioner, my first instinct was to rule out pathology. I ran all the ocular health tests—checked color vision, retinal responses, and every neurological variable I could think of. Everything came back normal.

But something about what he said wouldn't leave me. There was a truth in it I could feel, even if I couldn't find it in the data.

So, I trusted my gut.

I turned to his dad—someone I had built a strong relationship with over the years—and gently asked if I could speak with his son alone. Without hesitation, he said yes.

*When we were alone, I softened my voice and asked him, "Why do **you** think you're losing your color vision?"*

He shrugged. "I don't know."

I didn't push. I waited.

And then, slowly, he looked at me and said, "I just don't want to go to all these appointments anymore."

My heart cracked open.

He went on to describe how exhausted he was from being constantly therapized. Every week was filled with medical appointments—tests, evaluations, more therapy, more people trying to fix him. He didn't want to be fixed. He just wanted to ride his bike. Play outside. Be a kid.

*His words were so clear, so true, and so beautifully simple. His whole life had become a diagnostic journey—While his inner world had become **colorless.***

This wasn't a visual problem. This was a nervous system rebellion.

His brain was screaming, "Enough," and his visual system—the part of him that had been under constant scrutiny for years—responded the only way it could: by shutting down color.

And in that moment, I didn't try to correct him. I didn't prescribe anything new. I just told him the truth.

I explained how the nervous system sometimes goes into overload, and how vision is one of the most sensitive ways it communicates. I explained this to him like I would explain it to a colleague. And he understood. Completely. I saw him light up. I saw him smile and connect with me in a way I'll never forget.

That conversation changed everything.

From that day forward, the rigid black-and-white thinking began to soften. The spiral of overwhelm slowed. Something in his system had finally been acknowledged—not just managed, but deeply seen. He didn't need another strategy or intervention. He needed to feel witnessed. Validated. Met. What he had been calling "black and white" was, in truth, his nervous system begging for clarity, safety, and control in a world that felt too unpredictable. And in being seen, he could finally begin to release the grip. Before he left, I gently invited him to share this moment with his father—not just the clinical details, but the emotional truth—so that his healing could be received by both his own body and by the people who loved him most.

And that's what this work is about. It's not always about treatment. Sometimes, the most healing thing we can offer is presence. Stillness. Trust.

Sometimes, healing begins the moment someone believes you. And it did. That day, we didn't need more input. We needed resonance. And when we met his nervous system with understanding instead of intervention, the Field of Meaning softened—and color began to return.

Reflection for the Reader

Pause for a moment and consider this:

What if the symptoms we so often rush to correct—eye strain, avoidance of reading, postural shifts, "black and white" thinking—are not just neurological glitches or deficits . . . but emotional signals?

What if the visual system is not only receiving information from the outside world . . . but also broadcasting the unspoken truths of the inner world?

That child didn't need to "see better" in the conventional sense. He needed someone to see *him*—to recognize that his fixation on clarity was his nervous system's attempt to anchor in a world that felt blurred by emotional chaos. And once he was seen, his vision—on every level—began to regulate.

This is why the Neuro-Integrative Vision Model includes the Field of Meaning: not only to help patients see more clearly, but to help them rewrite what they've been unconsciously believing. To shift from protection to perception. From fear . . . to meaning.

The Neurology of Meaning-Making

Neurologically, this field is rooted in the ventral stream of visual processing, often referred to as the "What" pathway. This stream extends from the occipital lobe to the inferotemporal cortex and is responsible for object recognition, facial recognition, and the categorization of visual input.

However, meaning is not formed in isolation. It is shaped through neural convergence, particularly with:

- The amygdala, which assigns emotional relevance to visual input—often before we're aware of it
- The hippocampus, which encodes memory and contextual background to visual stimuli
- The prefrontal cortex, where beliefs, judgments, and social expectations are processed
- The limbic system, which integrates emotion, memory, and autonomic regulation

This network allows the visual system to go beyond recognition and into interpretation. It's not just about what we see—it's about what it means to us, and how that meaning informs our identity. What makes the Field of Meaning so profound—and sometimes so limiting—is how much of it operates beneath awareness. In my practice, this is often the layer accessed through emotional decoding, resonance-based prescribing, and what I now understand as the body's lens-language—the subconscious way it communicates its story through light. These meanings are not necessarily chosen. They are inherited, reinforced, and conditioned over time.

For instance:

- A child teased for reading slowly may internalize the belief that books equal failure—even after improving their skills.
- An adult who was shamed for their appearance may avoid mirrors, not because they cannot see themselves clearly but because what they see feels painful.
- A trauma survivor may walk into a room with perfect eyesight but perceive subtle facial expressions as dangerous based on past patterns.

In these examples, the visual system is not misperceiving objects—it is interpreting them through a lens of emotional history. That lens becomes subconscious, embedded in the nervous system, and difficult to access without intention. When the Field of Meaning is disrupted—through trauma, shame, or chronic invalidation—it can result in:

- Avoidance of visual tasks (reading, eye contact, mirrors)
- Hypervigilance or social anxiety
- Persistent internal narratives of inadequacy or invisibility
- Repetitive patterns of emotional reactivity to benign visual cues
- Difficulty integrating positive visual experiences

These disruptions often go unnoticed in clinical settings, especially when visual acuity appears normal. But patients report something deeper—an internal dissonance, a mistrust of what they see, or a belief that what they see is inherently flawed.

This isn't a refractive error. It's a perceptual wound.

Rewiring Meaning through Vision

The good news is that meaning is malleable. The visual system is remarkably adaptive, and the nervous system—given the right conditions—can rewire its emotional interpretations. When we introduce gentle lenses, tints, or structured visual therapy in an environment of emotional attunement, we create opportunities for meaning to shift. Because when perception becomes safe, interpretation becomes spacious. And in that space, a new reality begins to emerge—one where vision no longer reflects survival, but resonance.

- A child who once avoided books begins to approach them with curiosity after experiencing success with a new lens.
- An adult who felt disoriented in space begins to walk with calm after spatial integration work.
- A person who feared eye contact begins to soften in the presence of a safe gaze.

These shifts may seem subtle, but they represent profound reorganization of visual-emotional meaning.

Why This Field Matters

The Field of Meaning is where perception becomes personal. It is the space where the eye meets the heart—where vision is no longer just about recognizing objects, but about interpreting reality through the filter of who we believe we are.

In this field, vision does not simply reflect the external world—it mirrors the internal one. What we see is shaped by what we've lived: the unspoken wounds, the stories we've inherited, the emotions we've stored behind our eyes. A lens may sharpen clarity, but if what we see still evokes shame, fear, or grief, then vision has not truly healed.

This is where emotional imprint and visual function collide. It is also where the limbic field of the nervous system finds visual expression—where the unspoken becomes visible, and the invisible finally gets named. A person may have perfect tracking abilities yet still avoid reading because the page reminds them of years of failure. Another may avert their gaze—not due to a focusing issue, but because direct eye contact feels like exposure. A child may "refuse" to copy from the board not out of defiance, but because the space between the world and the self feels dangerous.

When we begin to uncover the emotional stories that vision holds, everything begins to shift. Sometimes subtly. Sometimes all at once.

Because once the body feels safe to process what has been held—once the nervous system is allowed to exhale—the entire visual system recalibrates. Posture realigns. Gaze softens. The environment feels less threatening. The world comes into view not just more clearly, but more compassionately.

This is the alchemy of meaning. When the emotional charge behind perception dissolves, the sensory system no longer needs to protect or distort. Vision opens.

In this way, we don't just improve visual performance—we open the possibility of a new reality. One where people not only see differently, but feel differently about what they see.

Because when meaning changes, the story changes.

And when the story changes, the *seer* is transformed. In the Field of Meaning, we don't just change how people see. We help them become safe enough to believe what they see—and to believe they belong in what they see.

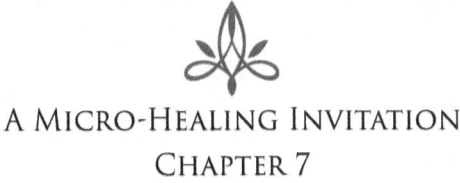

A MICRO-HEALING INVITATION
CHAPTER 7

The Field of Meaning: The Stories We See and the Beliefs That Shape Us

The visual system doesn't just record the world—it *interprets* it.

Every glance carries history.

Every moment of eye contact echoes a story.

The Field of Meaning is where sight becomes self-perception. It's where what you see becomes *what you believe about yourself.*

This field is shaped by more than cognition:

- It holds the memory of how others looked at you when you succeeded—or struggled.

- It reflects cultural messages, familial expectations, and the subtle imprint of trauma.

- It silently answers the question: *What does this say about me?*

Take a quiet breath. Then gently ask:

- Is there something I avoid seeing—not because I can't but because it carries meaning I haven't yet processed?

- Do I interpret certain faces, places, or pages through the lens of past judgment or shame?

These are not flaws in perception.

They are signs of a system doing its best to protect.

A Practice of Gentle Reinterpretation:

Choose one object that holds emotional charge—a photo, a journal, a mirror, a memory-laden item.

Look at it. Let your eyes settle. Breathe.

You don't need to change the story today. You just need to acknowledge it.

Silently offer:

"I am allowed to see this differently now. And I am allowed to see *myself* differently too."

The Field of Meaning is not fixed.

When perception shifts, so does possibility.

8
THE FIELD OF EXPRESSION

Being Seen. Seeing Others. Showing Up.

Vision isn't just about regulation. It's about radiance.

It's about what happens when the nervous system no longer asks, "Am I safe?" and instead begins to ask, "What can I share?" This is the shift from survival to presence. From contraction to contribution. And in the Neuro-Integrative Vision Model, it marks the arrival into relational coherence—the field where vision becomes connection.

This is the phase of life where joy gets loud. Where movement gets bold. Where expression becomes contagious.

And sometimes, that light comes through our children—teaching us what we've been afraid to remember.

Here's one of those stories.

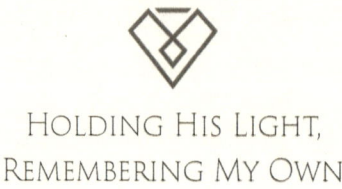

Holding His Light, Remembering My Own

My son Leo is pure light.

From the moment he was born, he radiated energy. Not the quiet, meditative kind—but the full-bodied, thunder-clapping, look-at-me-shining kind. He was the child who would burst into a room with wild joy, arms flung open, ready to be seen. Most of the time in nothing but his underwear!

And he wasn't afraid to take up space.

He laughed loudly. He played hard. He felt everything. And in his wake, he stirred something in me.

Something I wasn't expecting.

Because as much as I adored him—his sparkle, his magnetism—there were moments I felt myself . . . shrinking him.

Not out loud. Not with words. But in small, almost imperceptible ways.

"Shhh."

"Inside voice."

"Let's calm down."

"Not so much right now, honey . . . "

And every time, I could feel a flicker of dissonance in my body. As though a part of me knew: This isn't about him being too much. This is about me not knowing how to hold it.

I began to reflect. Where had I internalized the message that big joy was "too much"? That energy needed to be tamed? That exuberance had to be managed rather than celebrated?

It didn't take long to trace the thread.

I had been the child who felt deeply but learned to package it neatly. Who learned to perform instead of explode. Who made her intensity palatable so others wouldn't feel overwhelmed.

And suddenly, here was Leo—breaking all of that wide open.

His joy was an invitation to heal the part of me that believed I had to be smaller to be loved.

So I made a choice. Not a perfect one. Not a one-time epiphany. But a quiet, consistent promise to myself:

I will not dim his light just because I thought I needed to dim mine.

I began to let him be louder. Wilder. More himself. I began to let me feel the discomfort of joy that wasn't contained. And in that, something in both of us began to settle.

Leo is teaching me to hold radiance.

Not the polished kind—but the messy, exuberant, holy kind.

The kind that doesn't ask for permission.

The kind that isn't afraid to be loved exactly as it is.

And the more I allow him to take up space . . . the more space I find inside myself. Leo's unfiltered radiance reminded me of what most of us had to mask to survive. And in many patients, the Field of Expression isn't closed from pathology—it's closed from early messages that told them it wasn't safe to be fully seen.

Once the body has found grounding through space and posture, once attention has settled into clarity, and once meaning has begun to take root through visual-emotional interpretation, something remarkable begins to happen. The system no longer looks only inward. It turns outward. It begins to connect.

This is the moment when vision becomes relational. No longer just a tool for survival or self-orientation, it becomes a bridge between beings.

The gaze softens. The posture opens. The breath steadies. The visual system begins sending a new message—not just to the environment, but to the self: I belong here. I can connect. And the eyes, once used to scan for threat, begin to search for connection.

It is here—at this threshold—that vision shifts from function to presence.

Where seeing becomes a shared experience. Where being seen becomes a form of healing. Where expression begins not with words, but with the courage to let another in.

This is the emergence of the Field of Expression—the dimension of vision where safety, meaning, and self-awareness give rise to openness, engagement, and the most sacred human offering:

Here I am. And I see you too.

This is the part of vision that lets others know we are here. It is the field of being seen, of showing up, of making contact with the world not only through thought but through gaze, intention, and presence.

What Is the Field of Expression?

The Field of Expression is where the visual system intersects with social connection. It is the neural and energetic space where eyes become mirrors, transmitting and receiving subtle cues of emotion, safety, and belonging. In this field, the act of seeing becomes two-way. We are no longer observing—we are engaging. This is the point in the model where vision becomes relational energy. Not just looking—but meeting. Not just seeing—but sensing another nervous system with our own.

It includes:

- Eye contact (sustained, avoided, broken, or soft)
- Recognition and response to facial expressions
- Visual engagement and attunement in social interactions
- Mirroring of emotion through visual and motor pathways
- The interplay between gaze, vocal tone, and emotional regulation

This is why a single look can comfort or intimidate. Why someone's eyes can soften our body or, conversely, create tightness in our chest. Gaze becomes a language—one that is older than speech and deeper than words.

When this field is open and integrated, people tend to make eye contact naturally, feel present in conversation, and engage with others without overwhelm. When it is dysregulated, however, we may see social anxiety, avoidance of gaze, masking, emotional shutdown, or difficulty being seen—even when the desire for connection is present.

The Neurology of Expression

The Field of Expression relies on a beautifully complex system of neurological integration, drawing from both cortical and subcortical pathways that govern not only visual input but also social-emotional responsiveness.

Key areas include:

- The fusiform gyrus within the temporal lobe, which allows for facial recognition and decoding of subtle emotional expressions
- The anterior cingulate cortex, important for empathy, emotion regulation, and social monitoring
- The limbic system, particularly the amygdala, which assigns emotional tone to interactions and detects social safety or threat; this is the limbic lens, the filter that determines whether we show up fully—or retreat beneath the surface
- The cranial nerves, including the facial (7th cranial nerve), glossopharyngeal (9th cranial nerve), and vagus (10th cranial nerve), which coordinate micro-expressions, voice tone, and breath regulation

- The ventral vagal complex of the Polyvagal Theory, which activates social engagement when the nervous system perceives safety[3]

This field is a feedback loop. Our gaze affects our emotional state, and our emotional state affects our gaze. A person who feels threatened will avoid eye contact—not out of rudeness, but as a neurological withdrawal from perceived danger. A person who feels safe will soften their gaze, open their posture, and allow their voice to flow. In the Neuro-Integrative Vision Model, this is the convergence of meaning and presence. Where gaze becomes a gateway—not just for expression, but for repair.

Expression Is a Mirror of Regulation

In many clinical settings, we are taught to observe eye contact as a sign of social skill or confidence. But the deeper truth is that eye contact is a reflection of internal regulation. Poor or inconsistent gaze is not a behavior to be corrected—it is a message from the nervous system. When someone avoids your eyes, they may not be rejecting you—they may be trying to survive the intensity of being seen. For many, vision has been a channel of scrutiny or shame. To be seen is to feel exposed. So the eyes protect, even when the heart longs to connect.

And when we recognize this, we begin to shift our approach. We stop demanding connection and start creating conditions for it. We understand that expression is not only about teaching people to "make eye contact." It's about helping them feel safe enough to show

---

3   The neural pathways involved in expression—including the fusiform gyrus, anterior cingulate cortex, and cranial erves 7, 9, and 10—are well-documented in neuroscience literature (Kanwisher et al., 1997; Bush et al., 2000; Purves et al., 2001). These pathways are further shaped by the limbic system and ventral vagal complex, as explored in depth by LeDoux (2000) and Porges (2007).

up. Expression, then, is not a performance. It is a nervous system permission slip. And when we understand this, our work shifts from teaching behavior . . . to restoring trust.

The Role of Vision in Unlocking Expression

This is where vision therapy—and more broadly, the intentional use of lenses, tints, and visual-spatial interventions—becomes transformative. When we alter the visual input in ways that stabilize posture, balance spatial fields, or reduce visual overwhelm, we are not just changing clarity—we are changing access.

Access to voice. To gaze. To presence.

Patients who previously avoided interaction may begin to look up, to soften, to speak. Children on the spectrum may spontaneously vocalize. Adults who have felt chronically unseen may begin to meet the eyes of others with confidence.

This is not magic. It's coherence.

THE GIRL WHO SPOKE WITH HER EYES FIRST

She was seven years old, diagnosed with autism, non-verbal, and deeply withdrawn. Her mother had long given up on expecting verbal communication, but she brought her in to rule out any visual issues. What she didn't expect was what unfolded next.

The girl was guarded—averting gaze, shoulders high, breathing shallow. I didn't try to force interaction. I watched. I listened to her body. And then, I offered a soft therapeutic tint, one designed to reduce visual noise and stimulate the parasympathetic system.

She placed the lenses on. Her breathing changed. She stilled. And then she turned—slowly, deliberately—to look at her mother.

Their eyes locked.

Nothing was said, but everything was spoken.

Over the next weeks, she began using sounds. Then words. Her therapists called it a breakthrough. But what we witnessed was something even deeper: the return of safety in visual connection. The return of expression. The moment she made eye contact wasn't just about vision—it was about reentry. Into relationship. Into voice. Into being.

Why This Field Matters

Because this is the field where relational healing begins. Where gaze becomes a conduit for acceptance. Where people begin to feel witnessed.

This is not about social training—it's about nervous system restoration. It's about the right to take up space visually. To be seen not for performance, but for presence.

Expression Is Vision Coming Home

At its core, the Field of Expression teaches us something profound: vision is not just for taking in the world—it's also for offering ourselves to it. And when that offering is safe, sincere, and whole, we don't just express ourselves. We radiate. We become the vision. In the Neuro-Integrative Vision Model, the Field of Expression is the threshold before the deepest layer—the Field of Inner Vision. Because when presence is restored in the outer world, something sacred begins to stir within.

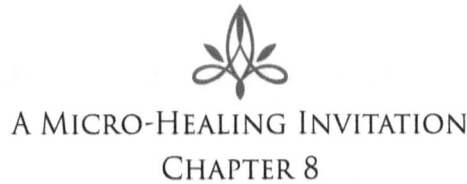

A Micro-Healing Invitation
Chapter 8

Field of Expression: Being Seen. Seeing Others. Showing Up.

There's a difference between looking and being seen—between observing and allowing yourself to show up.

The Field of Expression is where vision becomes relational. It's the place where the gaze becomes a bridge—not just a tool for attention, but a cue for connection.

For some, eye contact feels grounding. For others, it can feel vulnerable—too exposing, too much. This is not about social skills. It's about nervous system readiness.

Take a gentle moment to reflect:

- When I meet someone's gaze, does my body soften—or brace?

- Do I avoid eye contact—not out of disinterest, but because it feels too much to be witnessed?

- Have I ever been *truly* seen? And what happened in my body when it happened?

These are not personality traits. They're relational reflexes—deeply wired through past experiences of safety, trust, and attunement.

A quiet practice:

Sit in front of a mirror—not to judge or correct, but to witness.

Look into your own eyes. Just for a few breaths.

Then, with tenderness, say: "**It's safe to be seen. Even by myself.**"

Let that be enough.

You don't have to perform to be present.

You don't need perfect words or expressions to be real.

When your gaze becomes a place of safety—first for yourself—others will begin to feel it too.

Because when expression meets safety, the nervous system doesn't have to protect anymore.

It gets to connect.

9
THE FIELD OF INNER VISION

Where Emotion, Identity, and Soul Shape the Way We See

There's something different about treating your own child.

As a practitioner, I've worked with thousands of patients. I've seen trauma, regression, and incredible breakthroughs. I know the signs. I read the cues. But when it's your own son? The lens gets a little foggy.

My son Elliot has always been brilliant—intellectually curious, expressive, and deeply sensitive. He absorbs the world but with his mind and with his being. He notices subtleties that others don't— shifts in tone, unspoken emotions, undercurrents in a room. From a young age, I could feel how complex his inner world was.

And with that brilliance came a tenderness. A fragility around mistakes. He would crumple if he felt he'd gotten something wrong—not because he feared punishment, but because his own disappointment in himself was enough.

I knew this wasn't just about confidence or "self-esteem." This was neurological. Somatic. And, yes—emotional.

So I began observing him both as his mother and as a guide.

I watched how his body shifted when he tried to learn something new. I noticed how he held his breath. How his posture collapsed slightly when he got an answer wrong. I saw how much of his identity was wrapped around "getting it right."

But the most important moment didn't come from a test or a therapy session.

It came when I paused long enough to see him through a deeper frame.

Not just through the Four Circles as discussed in chapter 2—but through a Fifth.

That unseen, intuitive field where emotion, belief, and self-perception weave into vision. The space that holds trauma, yes—but also the soul's sensitivity. The why underneath the how.

Elliot's nervous system wasn't resisting information. It was defending against judgment.

The moment I realized that, everything shifted.

Instead of trying to bolster his confidence from the outside—through encouragement or praise—I began creating visual and emotional experiences that made his system feel safe to explore.

We played with lenses in gentle ways. I let him tell me what felt right. I created moments of wonder, not work. And I stopped trying to parent from performance. I started mirroring his inner world.

And in those small shifts, his system softened. He began to recover faster from mistakes. He stayed open longer during learning. He laughed more. It wasn't overnight. And it wasn't just from a lens.

It was from being seen.

Elliot is the reason I know the Field of Inner Vision is real. Because I didn't learn it from a patient.

I remembered it through him. Inner Vision is not something we diagnose. It's something we feel. Something we remember—through those we love, through those we serve, and through the moments that ask us to see with more than our eyes.

The Sensing, the Knowing, the Truth Beneath Sight

There is a kind of seeing that precedes clarity, precedes recognition, and even precedes awareness. It occurs before the brain has named an object, before thought has formed, and long before we've decided what we believe to be true. It's the kind of perception that lives in the body, in the subconscious, and in the energetic field surrounding every human experience. It's the way we know something without being able to explain why, and the way we feel a shift in a room before anyone speaks.

This is the Field of Inner Vision—the fifth and most subtle of the Neuro-Integrative Vision Model's five interconnected fields. It is the whisper underneath perception. The space where vision begins—not with light, but with readiness. Not with focus, but with felt truth. It is, in many ways, the most mysterious. It's the field where perception becomes instinct, where visual processing intersects with emotion and energy, and where science meets soul. Inner Vision does not operate through conscious logic or analytical reasoning. Instead, it arises from deep within the nervous system, often showing up as a felt sense of rightness, wrongness, safety, or truth—well before the eyes focus or the mind makes meaning.

Inner Vision is the realm of intuition, energetic resonance, limbic memory, and embodied knowing. It's the quiet but persistent awareness that something feels "off," even when everything looks normal. It's the ability to sense another person's presence without seeing them. It's the almost magical ability of some practitioners to select the perfect lens, not because of a measurable refraction, but because something about it feels aligned. Inner Vision is not imaginary. It is neurologically real. And yet, it is the most dismissed and misunderstood field of vision. And in the Neuro-Integrative Vision Model, it is the integrative field—the one that illuminates not just what is seen but how we are seen, and how we see ourselves.

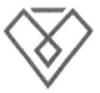

The Story of the Athlete Who Couldn't Read

She walked into my office like many others do—strong on the outside but hiding something deep beneath.

She was a professional athlete. Disciplined. Driven. Resilient. But when she sat down across from me, all of that fell away. Her eyes were wide. Her voice trembled.

She said, "I can't read."

I blinked. "What do you mean?"

"I mean," she said, "I can't read more than a sentence. I forget what I've read almost instantly. It's been like this for twenty years."

Twenty years.

She explained that at age fourteen, she had suffered a serious sports-related head injury—a skull fracture. That was the moment it began. Overnight, she went from being an "A" student to failing in school. Reading became a battlefield. Focus slipped through her fingers. She had seen top neurologists, optometrists, and sports medicine specialists. No one had helped.

She sustained more concussions over the years. Each one stole more of her clarity.

Still, she fought on. As a professional athlete, she had built an entire life around performance. But behind the victories, there was always this secret: she couldn't read.

Now, sitting in front of me two decades later, she asked me a question that stopped me cold:

"Can you fix me?"

It wasn't said with entitlement. It was said with desperation. With the kind of hope you don't want to admit you still have.

I began my assessment. What I found was staggering.

Her eye tracking was so disorganized, it couldn't even be scored on a standardized test—it was off the charts, quite literally. Her depth perception was virtually absent. Her binocular system showed massive suppression and instability. Every measure, every test, every reflex told the same story: this was a visual system in chaos. And yet, somehow, this young woman was performing at a professional level in her sport.

It defied everything we're taught to expect. By all clinical standards, her visual input should have been hindering her at every turn—disrupting timing, balance, coordination, and spatial orientation. But she had adapted in a way that was nothing short of extraordinary. Her brain had forged compensatory pathways, bypassed broken links, and re-mapped sensory terrain just to keep her in the game.

It was both awe-inspiring and heartbreaking. Because it meant no one had seen her clearly—not until now. Her outer performance had overshadowed her inner distress.

And yet, the moment we validated her truth—not just through testing, but through presence—her system began to remember how to heal.

We built her a custom program of vision therapy. Carefully. Compassionately. We rewired the neurological foundations that had been disrupted. We treated it not as an optical problem— but as a human one.

And she showed up. Every session. Every exercise. She brought the same tenacity that had made her successful in sport—and poured it into her healing.

And it worked.

Over time, her eye tracking improved from unscorable to the **99th percentile.** *Her depth perception returned. Her system stabilized. And—perhaps most astonishingly—she was able to read again.*

Really read.

Paragraphs. Pages. Books.

She wrote me this letter:

"As a teenager, I sustained a head injury following a sports-related skull fracture.

The injury caused me to have very poor reading comprehension. Overnight, I went from an "A" student to a failing student.

In the years following, I sustained multiple concussions, each of which caused more problems and made reading more and more difficult.

As a professional athlete, I had access to top physicians in their fields and was seen by neurologists, optometrists, and sports medicine physicians, but none of these doctors provided any solutions.

Twenty years after the initial injury, I was referred to Dr. Peddle. She immediately diagnosed me with severe post-traumatic vision syndrome from multiple closed-head injuries—telling me that my eyes were tracking so poorly it couldn't be scored on a standardized test, and that I had no depth perception.

Dr. Peddle provided me with a comprehensive treatment plan of vision therapy and executed that plan with a level of knowledge and expertise that I had not experienced anywhere else.

Thanks to Dr. Peddle, my eye tracking scores improved to the 99th percentile, I regained normal depth perception, and functionally—I was able to read again.

Dr. Peddle absolutely changed my life, and I could not be more thankful."

I read that letter often.

Because it reminds me that what we do in vision therapy is not just about sight.

It's about identity.

When someone loses the ability to read, they don't just lose function. They begin to forget who they are. They start to shrink. To doubt. To protect.

So when that capacity returns, it doesn't just change their performance.

It returns them to themselves. She didn't just regain her ability to read. She reclaimed the part of her that had been holding its breath for twenty years.

Practitioner's Reflection: When High Performance Masks Dysfunction

Elite athletes. High achievers. Perfectionists. They're the last ones anyone expects to have visual dysfunction.

But adaptation is powerful. The brain will build elaborate coping strategies to survive—especially when the stakes are high.

*Many of our highest-performing patients are functioning on **sophisticated compensations**, not integration.*

When someone is elite in one domain, their deficits in another are often ignored or misattributed—until they break.

As practitioners, we must learn to look beneath the surface.

Just because someone can play doesn't mean they can track.

Just because they "look fine" doesn't mean their system is safe.

Just because they cope doesn't mean they thrive.

This work isn't about enhancing performance for the sake of achievement.

*It's about restoring the nervous system so it can finally move from survival . . . to **self-expression.***

Inner Vision is what makes that leap possible. It is what tells the system: You're safe now. You can stop performing. You can begin becoming.

And that is where the true breakthroughs begin.

What Is Inner Vision?

The Field of Inner Vision refers to our capacity to perceive information through subtle, often subconscious, channels that don't rely on direct visual analysis. It is not the same as imagination, and it is not confined to abstract intuition. Rather, it is a body-based, neurologically encoded form of perception that draws on non-conscious visual pathways, emotional memory, and pre-verbal pattern recognition. This is the part of your system that notices shifts in light before your eyes adjust, that senses someone's emotional state before they speak, and that reacts to spatial or energetic fields in ways you can't quite explain. It is also the field your nervous system uses to read relational tone. To track resonance. To decide—in a flash—whether a moment holds danger . . . or potential.

Inner Vision becomes active in moments when logic fails to capture the full complexity of a situation—when you *just know* something is true, or when a subtle shift in posture or tone makes your whole body respond. Gut feelings, we like to call it. These are not metaphysical anomalies. They are the result of fast, subcortical processing that bypasses the conscious mind and emerges as a somatic signal—a change in breath, a tightening of the chest, a sudden calm, or an intuitive "yes."

This field is not separate from your visual system. It is its foundation. It is what allows the brain and body to respond to what is seen before you are aware that seeing has occurred. And perhaps more importantly, it is the field that gives context, tone, and truth to all the others. Inner Vision is the first field to awaken in infancy. And often, it is the last field we reclaim in healing. Because it asks us not to prove—but to trust.

The Neurology of Inner Vision

Although Inner Vision feels abstract, it is deeply grounded in well-established neuroanatomy. One of its key pathways is the tecto-pulvinar system, which sends information from the retina to the superior colliculus and pulvinar nucleus of the thalamus, bypassing the primary visual cortex entirely. This pathway allows visual stimuli to be processed subconsciously and almost instantaneously, activating emotional and motor responses before the brain has even formed a conscious image. It bypasses the mind—but not the self. And when this pathway is supported, patients don't just regain function. They regain *feeling*. They come home to the field of coherence.

The amygdala and insula play critical roles in this field, tagging sensory input with emotional valence and interoceptive awareness—how we perceive internal bodily states such as tension, warmth, or heart rate. The mirror neuron system, located primarily in the premotor cortex and inferior parietal lobe, allows us to attune to the emotional states of others through subtle facial cues and body movements, often without conscious recognition. Additionally, the right hemisphere, which specializes in nonverbal, holistic, and relational processing, plays a central role in synthesizing visual-spatial and emotional information into intuitive understanding.

When these systems work in harmony, a person may not be able to articulate why they feel the way they do—but their body and nervous system already know. The Field of Inner Vision explains why a certain room may feel heavy, why a child may recoil from a lens that looks optically neutral, or why a patient may burst into tears upon trying a prescription that feels emotionally "right." This is why so many transformations happen in silence. Because the Field of Inner Vision doesn't need words—it just needs resonance.

Why This Field Is Often Ignored

Despite being biologically valid and deeply influential, Inner Vision is frequently overlooked in both clinical and cultural contexts. In a society that prizes objectivity, data, and measurable outcomes, the subjective nature of this field is often viewed with skepticism or dismissed entirely. Children who perceive things others don't are labeled as distractible or overly sensitive. Adults who rely on their intuitive sense are often pressured to justify their insights with logic. Clinicians who choose a lens "by feel" may be criticized for not following standard protocols.

But ignoring this field does not erase it. What's dismissed by science is often what's most sacred in healing. And Inner Vision holds the very pulse of that sacred intelligence. In fact, suppressing Inner Vision often leads to heightened anxiety, disembodiment, and loss of self-trust. Patients whose systems are tuned into subtle energetic shifts are often gaslit by well-meaning professionals, told their sensitivities are imaginary or irrational. Over time, this leads to a dangerous disconnection from one's inner compass—the very system that was designed to protect and guide us long before science could explain it. It doesn't replace evidence—it completes it. It doesn't fight the mind—it invites the heart.

Reintegrating the Field of Inner Vision is not about abandoning science. It's about expanding our definition of what science includes. It's about honoring the full complexity of human perception—and giving space for what the nervous system knows before the conscious mind catches up.

Real-World Embodiment of Inner Vision

Clinically, this field shows up in powerful, often unexplainable ways. It's the patient who instantly relaxes when light levels are adjusted ever so slightly. It's the child who bursts into tears after trying on a lens that "shouldn't" make a difference—but does. It's the practitioner who chooses a prism or tint not because the numbers say it's right, but because their body, breath, and relational attunement guide them there. " I can finally breathe!" exclaimed one patient after sitting with a blue-violet tinted lens. These moments are not magical thinking. They are neurosensory integration at its most refined level. They are limbic re-patterning. They are nervous system permission. They are the visual system saying, *now I feel safe.*

One of the most profound examples I've experienced was with a young boy who barely spoke and rarely made eye contact. When I entered the room, he immediately looked away and buried his face in his hands. His mother assured me he could see, but said he was "highly sensitive." Instead of forcing engagement, I followed his cues. I introduced a subtle color filter—one I had used before to shift limbic responses through peripheral integration. He didn't reach for it or put it on. But as I moved it closer to his eyes, his posture softened. He looked toward me. Then, quietly, he said, "I feel better." That was all. But everything changed after that.

He wasn't responding to clarity. He was responding to **coherence**. Something in his system recognized the signal—and gave permission to emerge. Because Inner Vision doesn't wait for clarity—it responds to coherence. And in that moment, his body knew it was safe to be seen.

Inner Vision as the Integrative Field

While the other four fields of the Neuro-Integrative Vision Model—Body Vision, Focus, Meaning, and Expression—describe distinct dimensions of visual experience, the Field of Inner Vision is different. It is not one domain among equals. It is the connective tissue between them all.

Inner Vision orients the Field of Body Vision before we stabilize posture. It informs the Field of Focus before we filter attention. It shapes the Field of Meaning before we form belief. It attunes the Field of Expression before we connect to others. In this sense, Inner Vision acts as a guiding current, flowing through the entire system, preparing the terrain before any conscious action is taken. It is the pulse beneath presence. The tether between soul and sight. The first to feel, the last to be named.

When Inner Vision is active and integrated, the visual system becomes more than a sensory mechanism. It becomes a **mirror of truth**, a channel for self-recognition, and a gateway into embodied presence.

Inner Vision Is the Root of All Healing

To reconnect with this field is to remember something ancient and essential: that our body has always known how to see. This is the domain of the Limbic Balance Method—the terrain beneath behavior, beneath skill, where pattern becomes possibility, and energy becomes expression. Long before we were taught the alphabet chart or trained in refraction, we were reading energy, sensing shifts, tracking connection, and orienting to coherence. Reclaiming this field not only implies a neurological reorganization—it is a spiritual homecoming.

Inner Vision asks questions that don't appear on regular eye exams.

Can you trust what you feel before you explain it?

Can you move toward what resonates, even if no one else can see it yet?

Can you honor the wisdom that lives in your cells, even when the data isn't clear?

These observations highlight that vision is a complex, integrative function—woven into emotion, regulation, and perception. It is not localized to the eyes alone, but reflects the coordinated response of the entire system. Because vision, at its deepest level, is not about what we see. It's about *who we are when we are seen.*

A MICRO-HEALING INVITATION
CHAPTER 9

Field of Inner Vision: Seeing Yourself From Within
So much of life is spent training our eyes to look outward—to decode faces, read the room, stay "present."

But there is another kind of presence. One that turns gently inward. One that listens, not for words—but for truth.

The Field of Inner Vision is not about what you *see*.

It's about what you *sense*.

It's the space where intuition meets interoception.

Where insight rises before language.

Where you feel something is right—without needing to prove it.

Pause and reflect:

- When was the last time I *felt* a knowing before I could explain it?

- Do I give space to my intuition—or override it with logic?

- What if my body already knows what my mind is still trying to figure out?

This is not metaphysical.

It's neurological.

Your tecto-pulvinar system, your limbic brain, your interoceptive pathways—they've been listening all along.

A Mini Practice for Inner Vision Activation:
Gently close your eyes.

Place a hand on your chest, your belly, or your forehead—wherever feels right.

Ask yourself: "**What truth is waiting to be seen from within?**"

Then . . . wait.

Breathe.

Don't force an answer.

Let the body speak in sensation, stillness, or imagery.

Inner vision doesn't demand attention.

It waits for your willingness.

And when you begin to hear it, even faintly . . . the world outside often begins to shift too.

Not because it changed.

But because *you did.*

You were never meant to only see outward.

You were always meant to see in.

10

INTEGRATION OF
THE FIVE FIELDS

Where Vision Becomes Transformation

Vision is often mistaken for a checklist of observable skills—a measurable combination of acuity, tracking, attention, and eye alignment. It's categorized, scored, and treated as a discrete set of functions that either work well or don't. But when you truly begin to understand vision through the neuro-integrative lens, you come to realize that it is none of these things in isolation. Vision is not a skill. It is not a static function. It is not simply something you "do" with your eyes or even with your brain.

Vision is the embodied expression of your entire system—nervous, emotional, sensory, relational, and energetic—moving together in real time. It is a living, adaptive conversation between five distinct but deeply interconnected fields: Body Vision, Focus, Meaning, Expression, and Inner Vision. These fields do not operate in silos. They do not take turns. They move in fluid, dynamic relationship with one another, constantly shaping and reshaping the way you perceive, respond, and connect.

When these five fields come into alignment, vision stops being a task and becomes a portal—one that can open access to coherence, safety, creativity, and even transformation.

The Ocean, Not the Islands

In most traditional frameworks, visual function is taught and treated as a series of separate "skills" or deficits. Practitioners are trained to isolate variables: fix convergence here, train pursuits there, assess posture, diagnose processing. Each element is treated as an island—addressed with its own technique, protocol, or compensation strategy.

However, the Neuro-Integrative Vision Model reveals something different. It doesn't just name the islands—it makes visible the *ocean* that connects them. It shows us that **Body Vision** and **Focus** are not separate from one another, that the **Field of Meaning** cannot be disentangled from subconscious sensory input, and that **Expression**—through eye contact, voice, or presence—depends on deep coherence between emotion and perception. It shows us that **Inner Vision**, often invisible to the charts and graphs, is the current guiding the entire system.

These are not five steps in a linear process. They are five *currents* in a single living field. They rise and fall together. They echo, reinforce, and correct one another. And when one field becomes dysregulated, the others feel it—whether or not they show symptoms.

How the Fields Influence One Another

To understand the true power of integration, let's look at a single loop in the system.

Imagine a child whose Body Vision is unstable—perhaps due to early trauma, vestibular immaturity, or a disconnect between proprioception and visual grounding. When the body does not feel stable in space, the Field of Focus begins to strain. The nervous system, already in a heightened state of alert, must work harder to filter, track, and attend. Visual clutter becomes overwhelming. Attention fragments. The child becomes reactive.

This dysregulation spills over into the Field of Meaning. Now, every challenge is interpreted not just as difficult—but as unsafe. Beliefs begin to form: "I'm not good at this. I'm not smart. I'm not safe here." That internal narrative affects the Field of Expression. The child may avoid eye contact, withdraw socially, or appear angry or inattentive. And when that happens, the Field of Inner Vision— once vibrant and sensitive—goes quiet. The child no longer trusts what they feel, because the world keeps labeling it as wrong. The entire system folds inward.

From the outside, a clinician may see a child with no obvious "visual problem." Their acuity is 20/20. Their tracking is adequate. Their performance in structured tasks may even appear within normal limits. And yet, this child is struggling. They are overwhelmed, misdiagnosed, and misunderstood.

This is the cost of fragmentation. This is what happens when we treat the fields as separate.

But when we understand how these fields influence one another, we gain the power to shift everything—not by fixing the symptom, but by addressing the underlying coherence of the system.

Transformation Happens When the Fields Align

Integration is not about perfection. It is not about achieving flawless eye movements or eliminating all symptoms. True integration is about **coherence**—a state in which the five fields are in communication, in relationship, and in resonance with one another. It is a state where the nervous system no longer needs to protect or compensate because it feels safe to simply be.

When integration begins to unfold, we may see improvements in visual stamina, academic performance, or emotional regulation. But more often, we notice subtler signs of healing—things like a child breathing more deeply, standing taller, or spontaneously initiating eye contact. We see adults whose voices soften after years of guarded expression. We witness postural shifts, emotional releases, and even tears of recognition when a lens, a color, or a spatial shift unlocks something that words never could.

These are not miracles. They are signs that the five fields have begun to move together. That the person's perception is no longer fragmented. That their vision is not just functional—it is *alive*. Integration is not an end point—it is a return. To safety. To self. To seeing with the whole system again.

Your Role as a Guide to Integration

Whether you are a practitioner, a parent, a teacher, or someone on your own healing journey, your role is not to fix or direct the system.

Your role is to *witness* it. To hold space for it. To invite the fields back into conversation with one another.

Sometimes this happens through a carefully chosen lens—one that doesn't just correct vision, but initiates safety. Sometimes it begins with a question that no one else has asked, like "When did it first feel unsafe to see?" Sometimes it begins in silence, in the presence of someone who is willing to hold space for what the body knows but has never been allowed to express. Your gift is not in fixing what's broken. Your gift is in seeing what's hidden. In helping the nervous system feel safe enough to emerge.

This work is sacred. And it is often quiet. But its effects are profound.

When a person experiences integration—when the five fields begin to align—they often describe it not as improvement, but as *return*. They say things like, "I feel like myself again," or "I didn't know how lost I was until I landed." That landing isn't always dramatic. Sometimes, it's as subtle as a breath. As quiet as a gaze. But once it happens—you know.

Vision as Liberation

At its highest level, the Neuro-Integrative Vision Model offers more than clinical outcomes or performance gains. It offers a new paradigm. It invites us to see vision as not only a sensory system, but as a mirror—a mirror of emotional truth, subconscious patterning, nervous system balance, and spiritual presence.

When the five fields integrate, vision becomes more than function. It becomes transformation. It becomes the key that unlocks regulation, resilience, and relational connection. It becomes the bridge between trauma and healing, between protection and presence, between fear and full participation in life. It becomes the moment a person stops surviving . . . and starts seeing themselves as whole.

And perhaps most powerfully, it becomes a path of liberation—a way to return home to the truth of who we are, how we feel, and what we are here to see.

The Girl Who Couldn't Be Touched

She was eight years old when her mother brought her in. Quiet, withdrawn, almost motionless in the chair. Her posture was curled in, legs crossed tight beneath her, hands tucked under her thighs like she was trying to disappear. She wouldn't make eye contact, wouldn't speak, and every time I moved even slightly in her direction, she flinched. Her mother explained she'd been like this for years. "She's afraid of being touched," she said, her voice tight with exhaustion. "Not just physically—but visually. She doesn't even want anyone looking at her. Not even me."

They'd tried everything. Pediatricians. Occupational therapy. Counseling. "She's fine," they were told. "She'll grow out of it. She's just shy." But her mother knew better. Her daughter was pulling further and further away from life.

*I began my assessment—not with the chart, but with obser-vation. Her **Body Vision** was clearly dysregulated; she didn't know where she was in space and couldn't tolerate open envi-ronments. Her **Field of Focus** was scattered; her eyes would dart and then freeze, as if the very act of attention was a threat. She couldn't hold convergence. Couldn't track. Couldn't sit still long enough to try.*

*And yet, what stood out the most was her gaze. It wasn't absent—it was guarded. As if her **Field of Meaning** had encoded the world as something unsafe, and vision itself had become a channel of vulnerability. Her **Expression** was blocked; her face had no animation, and her voice was barely audible. And her **Inner Vision**? Silent. There was no resonance in the room—no flicker of curiosity, no subconscious shift. Her system had gone offline.*

She didn't need to learn how to read letters on a chart. She needed to come home to herself.

So I started where her nervous system lived: with safety. I introduced a lens—not for clarity, but for orientation. A gentle yoked prism to stabilize her visual midline. I dimmed the lights. Shifted the chair slightly to give her more peripheral support. I had her mother sit behind her instead of beside her—small adjustments to the field, but with big messages to her body: You are not being watched. You are safe to settle.

Over the weeks that followed, I didn't push. I tracked the tiny signs of reintegration. First, her feet began to touch the ground instead of curling up. Then she sat a little taller. In one session she reached out to touch a toy on the table—her first sponta-neous action in my presence. She still didn't speak. But her **Body Vision** *was waking up.*

As the fields began to shift, I introduced a light-filtering tint— just enough to lower her arousal without dulling her presence. She began to make fleeting eye contact. Then longer. Then she smiled—once. Quiet, quick. But it was there. Her **Field of Focus** *improved. Her saccades became smooth. Her ability to shift attention began to emerge.*

By the third month, she looked me in the eye and said, "I don't feel dizzy anymore." That was the first sentence she'd spoken in the office.

Over the next few months, I watched her blossom. We worked on posture, convergence, figure-ground, and meaning-making through games. She didn't just tolerate eye contact—she started initiating it. Her **Expression** *returned, not because we taught it, but because we made it safe. She began using her voice. Asking questions. Leaning forward instead of curling in.*

And the moment I knew her **Inner Vision** *had come back online?*

She interrupted a session to ask me, "Do you think maybe my eyes got scared before I did?"

I paused. Stunned by the depth of her awareness.

"Yes," I said. "I think your whole system was protecting you the best way it knew how."

She nodded and then replied, "But I think they're okay now."

That moment—more than any test result—told me she was healing. That is the work of integration. Not just correcting vision—but restoring trust. In space. In connection. In self.

Integration is not a destination. It is a rhythm. A remembering. When the five fields move together, vision becomes more than sight. It becomes presence. It becomes possibility.

And in that presence—we don't just see differently. We live differently. And that, more than anything else, is what this model was built for.

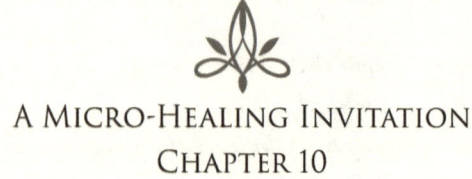

A MICRO-HEALING INVITATION
CHAPTER 10

Integration of the Five Fields

Wiring Vision Back into Wholeness
The five fields of vision—**Body, Focus, Meaning, Expression, and Inner Vision**—are not isolated skills.

They are a living system.

A network of perception, safety, emotion, and attention.

Each one shapes the others.

Each one carries its own wisdom.

But integration?

That's when vision becomes transformation.

Integration doesn't mean perfection.

It means coherence.

It's when your body, brain, and field stop working in fragments—and start moving in harmony.

It's when your system no longer has to guard one part while overcompensating with another.

It's when vision becomes a whole-body experience again.

A quiet reflection:

- Which field do I feel most at home in? Where do I feel naturally resourced or steady?

- Which field feels more distant, tender, or hard to access right now?

- What might my nervous system be trying to protect by holding that field back?

A Mini Practice for Field Reconnection:

1. Draw five simple circles on a blank page.

2. Label them:
   - Body
   - Focus
   - Meaning
   - Expression
   - Inner Vision

3. Place your hand over your heart or belly and ask, "Which field is asking for care today?"

4. Let the answer emerge—not through logic, but through sensation.
   Maybe a color comes to mind. A word. A gesture. A breath.
   Doodle. Move. Write. Breathe into it.

This is how integration begins—not in fixing everything at once, but in listening deeply to the part that's ready to rejoin the whole.

Because when vision becomes integrated, you don't just see differently—you begin to feel like yourself again.

11
Becoming the Vision

Living, Guiding, and Embodying the Five Fields

You've now walked through the five fields. You've explored vision as more than clarity—as something deeply sensory, emotional, subconscious, and sacred. Along the way, you've felt the threads of the nervous system, the influence of trauma, the presence of intuition, and the possibility of transformation. And now, you arrive at the most important truth of all:

You are not separate from this model.

You *are* the model.

You live inside it. You breathe through it. You carry it in the way you observe others, hold space, interpret the world, and even make decisions about your own life. This is not a theory you apply from the outside—it is a lens you embody from the inside out.

To become the vision is to release the need to "fix" people's sight and instead support them in returning to it. It's the shift from treating parts in isolation to recognizing the entire system in motion. It's the moment you stop reaching for clarity as something external, and instead begin to allow clarity to emerge from the body, from safety, from coherence.

This model isn't just a clinical tool. It's a life practice. It's a transformation. A way of being. And when you begin to live it, your entire way of seeing the world begins to shift.

The Model Is Not a Tool. It's a Transformation.

When you live this model, you don't just become a better practitioner—you become a more attuned human being. You become more present in your own body. You begin to trust the sensory whispers that arise before language. You listen to the signals beneath the symptoms. You begin to see your patients, clients, children, or loved ones not through a diagnostic framework, but through the real-time fluidity of their field state.

You stop asking, "What's wrong with this person?"

And instead begin to ask, "What is their vision trying to reveal?"

This simple shift changes everything. It brings compassion into precision. It transforms reaction into presence. It allows you to offer the kind of attuned support that creates safety— for the entire system.

You begin to feel what is open, what is collapsed, what is straining to stay functional, and what is quietly asking to be held. You learn to see more than the behavior or the symptom, but the field behind it.

Practices for Living the Model

If you are wondering how to begin living this work—not just understanding it, but *inhabiting* it—start here. Let these be invitations, not instructions.

1. Practice Noticing the Five Fields in Yourself

Each day, take a moment to check in with your own fields. It doesn't have to be formal—just an honest inquiry.

- **Body Vision**: Do I feel grounded in space today, or am I floating above myself?
- **Focus**: What feels clear in my world? What feels scattered, disorganized, or hard to track?
- **Meaning**: What unconscious story am I assigning to this experience, this person, or this emotion?
- **Expression**: Do I feel safe to be seen right now? Do I feel safe to show up as myself?
- **Inner Vision**: Is there something I'm sensing that doesn't have language yet?

You don't need to fix or force anything. This is not a diagnostic scan. It's an act of relational self-awareness—a way of building fluency in your own nervous system.

2. See Others through the Five Fields

Whether you are working with a patient, sitting with your child, or listening to a friend, practice seeing through the fields.

- Is this person's **Body Vision** giving them a sense of safety in the room—or are they fighting gravity?
- Is their **Focus** field overwhelmed or under-responsive?
- Are they interpreting this moment through a **Meaning** field shaped by fear, shame, or conditioning?
- What are they trying to **Express** but don't yet feel safe enough to say?
- What might their **Inner Vision** be whispering that they've learned to ignore?

This kind of vision makes you not just a healer—but a witness. And witnessing is one of the most powerful healing forces we have.

3. Ask Better Questions

Shift the conversation from outcome-based questions to ones that invite felt experience and body-based knowing.

Instead of, "What do you see?" try,

- "What do you feel in your body when you look at this?"
- "What shifts when you breathe and allow your eyes to rest?"
- "Where do your eyes go when you feel overwhelmed?"
- "Does this lens make your system feel more at ease, even if you can't explain why?"

These questions bypass the need for performance and open the door to nervous system truth. They allow vision to speak—not from the cortex, but from coherence.

4. Trust the Subtle

As you become the vision, you will begin to notice the smallest shifts: a change in breath, a softening of the jaw, a flicker of clarity in the eyes. These moments matter. Trust them.

You are allowed to trust goosebumps.

You are allowed to trust stillness.

You are allowed to trust when a child sighs and lands in their body for the first time all day.

You are allowed to trust your intuition when it tells you a shift has occurred—before the test results say so.

This is vision speaking through the nervous system. And you are attuned enough to hear it.

Becoming the Vision Is a Lifelong Practice

There will be days when you feel aligned—when your perception is clear, your nervous system is grounded, and your presence is expansive. And there will be days when your own fields feel fragmented, overstimulated, or offline. This is not failure. This is the work. This is the dance of living inside a body, inside a world that is constantly asking for adaptation.

Vision is not a fixed skill.

It is a living, breathing dialogue between your body, your brain, your soul, and the field around you.

When you live this way, you become more than a provider.

You become a guide. A messenger. A mirror.

You help others remember what it feels like to be seen with reverence—and to see themselves with love.

Because the truth is: the vision was never broken.

It was never lost.

It was simply waiting.

Waiting for someone to slow down.

To pay attention.

To listen.

And now . . .

You are that someone.

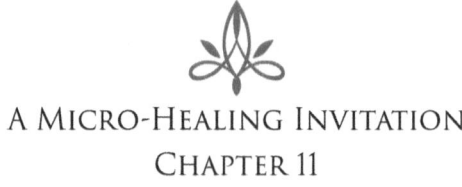

A Micro-Healing Invitation
Chapter 11

Becoming the Vision

This final chapter invites you to shift—from understanding vision to embodying it. Because transformation doesn't come from knowledge alone. It comes from integration. From alignment. From living what you now know to be true.

You are no longer a passive observer.

You are a participant. A seer. A guide.

Your visual system is not a tool to correct—it's a language to live by.

Reflection Prompts:

- Since beginning this journey, what have you started to *see differently*—in yourself, your work, and your relationships?

- Where are you being called to see more clearly . . . or more compassionately?

- What would it mean to live not just with sight but with aligned inner vision?

Final Integration Practice

Close your eyes.

Take a few slow, intentional breaths.

Now, imagine a soft light—not outside of you, but behind your eyes. This is your inner lens—quiet, knowing, precise.

Let it expand gently through your breath, your spine, your voice.

Ask yourself:

If my perception were fully aligned with truth—how would I move today?

How would I speak? Listen? Choose?

What would I no longer ignore?

What would I allow myself to see?

When you're ready, open your eyes. Not only to the world—but to yourself.

You are not here to fix vision.

You are here to become it.

You are the model.

You are the guide.

You are the vision that's been waiting to be seen.

Epilogue

The Light Has Always Been There

You haven't just read a book—you've journeyed back to something your body always knew. A return to what your body knows, and your soul doesn't forget.

Page by page, field by field, story by story, you've reclaimed something sacred—your ability to see from within. Not only to take in the world around you, but to witness it from the inside out. You've remembered that vision isn't only about what's visible. It's about what's *true*. And what's true has always lived within you.

This journey was never about fixing what's broken.

It was about softening into what's always been whole.

It was about seeing with your nervous system. Feeling with your gaze. Trusting your body's knowing before the mind had words for it.

When you make it to this point, you've probably realized—this wasn't just about vision therapy.

Yes, you've read clinical stories. You've seen case transformations. You've learned how a lens or prism can shift the nervous system, how color can open a portal, and how safety often precedes speech, movement, or learning.

But beneath it all, this book was always about *seeing*. Not just with the eyes. Not just with the brain. But with the self.

Because vision is more than clarity. It's more than acuity. It's more than the ability to recognize a letter on a chart.

Vision is relationship.

It's how we orient to the world. How we know where we are in space. How we regulate ourselves in chaos. How we perceive others—and how we believe they perceive us.

When I began my career, I thought I was learning how to help people "see better." And I was.

But what I didn't know then—what I've come to understand now—is that I was also learning how to help people return to themselves. I was learning to recognize the silent ways we disconnect, and the subtle tools that can guide us back.

Lenses.

Color.

Prism.

Attention.

Trust.

These aren't just interventions. They are *invitations*.

Each one whispers: *You're safe now. You can come forward. It's okay to be seen.* And that invitation isn't just for the patients. It's for us.

Because once you begin to see through this lens—once you stop separating science from soul—you begin to feel something shift inside you too. You start noticing what feels off. You start sensing what's ready to change. You start seeing yourself with a new kind of clarity—not through judgment, but through compassion.

So if you've felt something stir while reading this, let it. If a story brought up emotion, allow it to rise. If your body responded to a sentence, a metaphor, a memory—trust that response.

This is what happens when vision becomes integrative. It touches more than just the eyes. It reaches the nervous system. The story. The self.

And you don't need to be a doctor or a therapist to feel that. You only need to be *ready.*

So now we reach the end—but not really.

Because what I hope is that this book becomes a doorway for you. A gentle knock from the part of you that's been waiting to be seen more fully—whether that's as a healer, a parent, a patient, or a person who's simply ready to reclaim their own light.

And if that's you?

Welcome.

You're not just looking through the lens anymore. You're becoming it. **See on.** The world is waiting for your gaze.

And so—if you're ready to return to yourself,

to trust what your body sees,

to witness what your nervous system already knows...

Just remember:

The light has always been there.

Appendix A

The Neuro-Cognitive Model

Sources to learn more about the Neuro-Cognitive model include:

Dorsal Stream
Kravitz, D. J., Saleem, K. S., Baker, C. I., Ungerleider, L. G., & Mishkin, M. (2013). "The ventral visual pathway: An expanded neural framework for the processing of object quality." *Trends in Cognitive Sciences*, 17 (1), 26–49.

Ventral Stream
Grill-Spector, K., & Weiner, K. S. (2014). "The functional architecture of the ventral temporal cortex and its role in categorization." *Nature Reviews Neuroscience*, 15 (8), 536–548.

Pulvinar Nucleus
Arcaro, M. J., Pinsk, M. A., & Kastner, S. (2015). "The anatomical

and functional organization of the human visual pulvinar." *Journal of Neuroscience*, 35 (27), 9848–9871.

Superior Colliculus
Krauzlis, R. J., Lovejoy, L. P., & Zénon, A. (2013). "Superior colliculus and visual spatial attention." *Annual Review of Neuroscience*, 36, 165–182.

Reticular Activating System (RAS)
Moruzzi, G., & Magoun, H. W. (1949). "Brain stem reticular formation and activation of the EEG." *Electroencephalography and Clinical Neurophysiology*, 1(1–4), 455–473.

Parietal Lobe
Andersen, R. A. (1997). "Multimodal integration for the representation of space in the posterior parietal cortex." *Philosophical Transactions of the Royal Society B: Biological Sciences*, 352 (1360), 1421–1428.

Cerebellum
Kheradmand, A., & Zee, D. S. (2011). "Cerebellum and ocular motor control." *Frontiers in Neurology*, 2, 53.

Appendix B

Scientific Foundations Behind the Intuition

While the stories and clinical reflections in this book are deeply expe-
riential, they are grounded in a growing body of scientific literature
that validates what many of us have long sensed: the nervous system
responds to visual input in ways that extend far beyond clarity.

Below are studies and references that support the clinical use
of low-powered lenses and yoked prisms, especially in the context of
nervous system regulation, posture, spatial orientation, and emotional
integration:

Yoked Prisms

- **Kapoula Z, et al. (2007).** "Effects of visually induced
  postural sway and yoked prism glasses on posture and visual
  stabilization." *Vision Research.*
  - » Demonstrated that yoked prisms can significantly
    influence postural alignment, especially in patients with
    visually induced instability.

- **Rossi P, et al. (2015).** "The effect of yoked prisms on the perception of visual vertical and spatial orientation." *Frontiers in Psychology.*
  - » Found that yoked prisms effectively shift perceived midline and enhance spatial orientation, particularly in populations with spatial neglect.

Low-Powered Lenses

- **Grisham JD, et al. (1993).** "The effect of low plus lenses on reading performance in children with learning problems." *Journal of Behavioral Optometry.*
  - » Showed that low-plus lenses improved reading efficiency and comfort in children experiencing near point visual stress.

Integrative Vision and Neural Pathways

- The role of the **pulvinar nucleus**, **superior colliculus**, and **reticular activating system** in visual attention and trauma responses is well documented in neuroanatomy literature.
- These structures mediate subconscious filtering and orienting—anatomically validating the intuitive and somatic experiences described throughout this book.

These studies, alongside thousands of clinical case reports from behavioral optometrists worldwide, reflect what we've always known: vision is not just seen—it is *felt*. And sometimes, the smallest lens can open the biggest doorway to change.

REFERENCES

Andersen, R. A., & Cui, H. (2009). "Intention, action planning, and decision making in parietal-frontal circuits." *Neuron*, 63 (5), 568–583.

Culham, J. C., & Valyear, K. F. (2006). "Human parietal cortex in action." *Current Opinion in Neurobiology*, 16 (2), 205–212.

Garcia-Rill, E. (2015). "Waking and the Reticular Activating System." Academic Press.

Goodale, M. A., & Milner, A. D. (1992). "Separate visual pathways for perception and action." *Trends in Neurosciences*, 15 (1), 20–25.

Koziol, L. F., Budding, D. E., et al. (2014). "Consensus paper: The cerebellum's role in movement and cognition." *The Cerebellum*, 13 (1), 151–177.

May, P. J. (2006). "The mammalian superior colliculus: Laminar structure and connections." *Progress in Brain Research*, 151, 321–378.

Moruzzi, G., & Magoun, H. W. (1949). "Brain stem reticular formation and activation of the EEG." *Electroencephalography and Clinical Neurophysiology*, 1 (1–4), 455–473.

Saamann, Y. B., & Kastner, S. (2011). "Cognitive and perceptual functions of the visual thalamus." *Neuron*, 71 (2), 209–223.

Schmahmann, J. D., & Sherman, J. C. (1998). "The cerebellar cognitive affective syndrome." *Brain*, 121 (4), 561–579.

Shipp, S. (2003). "The functional logic of cortico–pulvinar connections." *Philosophical Transactions of the Royal Society B: Biological Sciences*, 358 (1438), 1605–1624.

Sparks, D. L. (2002). "The brainstem control of saccadic eye movements." *Nature Reviews Neuroscience*, 3 (12), 952–964.

Ungerleider, L. G., & Mishkin, M. (1982). "Two cortical visual systems. In D. J. Ingle, M. A. Goodale, & R. J. W. Mansfield (Eds.) Analysis of Visual Behavior." (pp. 549–586). MIT Press.

ABOUT THE WRITING PROCESS

While writing *Becoming the Vision*, I knew I wasn't just sharing a clinical model—I was translating a way of seeing the world that had been evolving inside me for years. The stories, insights, and framework of the Neuro-Integrative Vision Model are all deeply personal and original to my own clinical and healing journey.

To help bring that vision fully to life on the page, I collaborated with an editorial partner who supported me in refining the language, enhancing structure, and making sure my voice, energy, and message could be felt clearly by a broad audience. Every case study, concept, and transformation came from my own experience. The editorial process simply helped shape the rhythm and resonance of my words—so they could reach more people, more powerfully.

Acknowledgments

Writing *Becoming the Vision* has been a transformative journey, one that would not have been possible without the inspiration and encouragement of many remarkable individuals.

To my husband, Dr. Jeff Speers, and children, Elliot and Leo, thank you for your support, inspiration, and love. To my parents and sister, who unknowingly helped me form the fields throughout my childhood and inspired me to find my true inner vision.

To all my colleagues in the field of vision therapy—your unwavering commitment and resilience are a constant source of inspiration. Each day, you challenge conventional norms, advocating for transformative approaches that profoundly impact patients' lives. Your dedication, often in the face of skepticism, exemplifies the remarkable work that continues to advance our field.

To Dr. Robert Sanet, who provided not only the scaffolding upon which I built this manuscript but also the mentorship and encouragement to take this leap. To Drs. Nancy Torgerson, Stelios Nikolakakis, and Vi Tu Banh—thank you for believing in me before I truly believed in myself. Your unwavering encouragement in my darkest moments has been instrumental in my journey, providing the confidence and guidance needed to pursue this path.

To Krista Clive-Smith—thank you for planting the seed that would become *Becoming the Vision*. I didn't know this seed was growing deep inside me until it burst through with cosmic force and light, needing to be told. To my editor, Amy Valentine, whose insights and guidance refined my thoughts and words, bringing clarity to complex ideas.

To all my patients, whose resilience and trust have been instrumental in shaping the concepts within these pages. Your journeys have provided invaluable insights and have been central to the development of this work.

Finally, to all who believe in the power of vision to heal and transform—this book is for you.

ABOUT THE AUTHOR

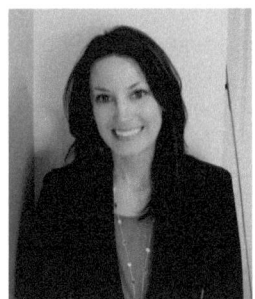

Dr. Angela Peddle, OD, is an internationally recognized neuro-optometrist, educator, and the creator of the Neuro-Integrative Vision Model™—a groundbreaking framework that weaves together neuroscience, developmental vision therapy, subconscious processing, and emotional regulation.

Her work helps individuals of all ages move beyond traditional notions of "20/20," guiding them to access the deeper intelligence of their visual system—where clarity, embodiment, and healing intersect.

As the co-founder of Elite Vision Therapy Centre in Toronto, Ontario, Dr. Peddle has led thousands of patients—ranging from children with developmental challenges to adults recovering from trauma—through life-changing care. Her innovative lens and light-based protocols have redefined what's possible in vision rehabilitation.

Inspired not only by science but also by her lifelong love for music and art, Angela brings a deeply creative lens to her work. She has spent years bridging the intuitive and the analytical—piecing together her passion for meaning, harmony, and depth with her clinical mastery.

Through her global education platform, Neuro Visual Consultants, she mentors and trains optometrists and therapists around the world, helping professionals expand both their clinical precision and intuitive insight.

In *Becoming the Vision*, Dr. Peddle brings decades of expertise into a powerful offering that is both scientific and sacred. She invites readers to reimagine vision not as a score, but as a living system—one that carries memory, emotion, identity, and the possibility for profound transformation.

Because the way we see isn't just what we look at—

It's how we know ourselves.